In Your Own Time
How western medicine controls the start of labour and why this needs to stop

Dr Sara Wickham

In Your Own Time: How western medicine controls the start of labour and why this needs to stop

Dr Sara Wickham

Published 2021 by Birthmoon Creations
Avebury, Wiltshire
© 2021 Sara Wickham
www.sarawickham.com

Sara Wickham has asserted her moral right to be named as the author of this work in accordance with the Copyright, Designs and Patents Act of 1988.

ISBN: 9781914465024
Also available as an e-book

Cover design by Sam Aalam

All rights reserved. No part of this book may be reproduced or transmitted in any form by any means for any commercial or non-commercial use without the prior written permission of the author. This book is sold subject to the condition that it shall not, by way of trade and otherwise, be lent, resold, hired out or otherwise circulated without the publisher's prior consent in any form or binding or cover other than that in which it is published and without a similar condition being imposed upon the subsequent purchaser.

This book offers general information for interest only and does not constitute or replace individualised professional midwifery or medical care and advice. Whilst every effort has been made to ensure the accuracy and currency of the information herein, the author accepts no liability or responsibility for any loss or damage caused, or thought to be caused, by making decisions based upon the information in this book and recommends that you use it in conjunction with other trusted sources of information.

Acknowledgements

This book wouldn't exist if it hadn't been for two people who gave up some of their summer to edit it as I wrote (even though they are two of the busiest people I know) so that we could publish it when it would be needed most. Nadine Edwards and Julie Frohlich bring completely different and (much to my benefit) totally complementary skills and this book is so much better for their input. Thank you both, with special thanks to Nadine for editing and support above and beyond the call of duty and to Julie for writing the foreword.

My husband Chris supports me and my work in a million ways, not least of which is checking all the references and making the electronic versions of my books work. I also want to acknowledge the long-term help and support of Mavis Kirkham, who midwifed me through the PhD which was a huge stepping stone in my work on induction of labour, and who has been on the journey with me ever since.

A flock of other equally wonderful friends and colleagues have also supported the creation of this book, in many ways. They have nourished me with meals, wine, stories, research and encouragement. They have shared their publishing, proofreading and technical knowledge and skills with me. Some have sent chocolate, let me write in corners of their homes and listened while I worked out how to turn five books into one. These fabulous people include (but are not limited to) Lucyann Ashdown, Beverley Beech, Gill Boden, Amanda Burleigh, Penny Champion, Emma Mills, Jo Murphy-Lawless, Kim Osterholzer, Rachel Reed, Emma Rose and Debbie Willett, and I am immensely grateful to you all.

Finally, a huge thank you to those who have allowed me to share their words and stories, and to you, for caring enough about women, babies, families and birth to read this book.

About the Author

Dr Sara Wickham PhD, RM, MA, PGCert, BA(Hons) is a midwife, author, speaker and researcher who works independently; speaking, writing, teaching online courses and workshops, consulting and creating resources for health professionals, birth workers, writers and others.

Sara's has lived and worked in the UK, the USA and New Zealand, edited three professional journals and lectured in more than twenty-five countries. This is her eighteenth book.

You can find and follow Sara online at her website, www.sarawickham.com, where she writes a blog and offers a free monthly newsletter sharing birth-related information.

Sara is also on Instagram as @DrSaraWickham.

Also by Sara Wickham

Anti-D Explained
Anti-D in Midwifery: panacea or paradox?
Appraising Research into Childbirth
Birthing Your Placenta (with Nadine Edwards)
Group B Strep Explained
Inducing Labour: making informed decisions
Midwifery Best Practice (volumes 1-5)
Sacred Cycles: the spiral of women's wellbeing
Vitamin K and the Newborn
What's Right for Me? Making decisions in pregnancy and childbirth
101 Tips for planning, writing and surviving your dissertation

Contents

FOREWORD 1

INTRODUCTION 5

1. THE ADVANTAGES OF THE WAITING DAYS 11

    THE VALUE OF RIPENING 12
    THE HORMONAL ORCHESTRA 13
    AVOIDING THE PROBLEMS OF BEING BORN TOO EARLY 16
    OTHER BENEFITS OF SPONTANEOUS LABOUR FOR BABIES 21
    ADVANTAGES OF SPONTANEOUS LABOUR FOR WOMEN 22
    WIDER BENEFITS, NESTING AND THE TIME OF ZWISCHEN 25
    SUMMARISING THE BENEFITS 27

2. WHY DOESN'T EVERY WOMAN GET TO BIRTH IN HER OWN WAY? 29

    THE MILLION POUND QUESTIONS 30
    WHY IDEAS MATTER 32
    HOW BIRTH MOVED FROM HOME TO HOSPITAL 32
    THE TECHNOCRATIC PARADIGM 34
    WOMEN AREN'T MACHINES 37
    SEPARATION DOES MORE HARM THAN GOOD 40
    BABIES AREN'T END PRODUCTS 42
    BIRTH AS RISKY BUSINESS 44
    RISK MANAGEMENT LACKS LOGIC 46
    THE RISKS OF THE OBSTETRIC APPROACH 47
    BIRTH AND TIME 49

3. GUIDELINES, EVIDENCE AND LISTENING TO WOMEN 53

    THE 'OFFER' OF INDUCTION 54
    WHY 'THE NORM' MATTERS 57

- THE PROBLEMS WITH THE DRAFT GUIDELINE 58
- WOMEN'S EXPERIENCES OF INDUCTION 61
- WHY DO SOME WOMEN DISLIKE INDUCTION SO MUCH? 63
- WHAT DO MIDWIVES AND BIRTH WORKERS THINK? 65
- WHAT SHOULD WE DO ABOUT IT? 68
- WHERE DO WE GO FROM HERE? 72

4. DUE DATES, WINDOWS AND WHY THE COMPUTER SHOULDN'T DECIDE 73

- WHERE'S THE PROBLEM? 74
- THE HISTORY OF THE DUE DATE 76
- FIXED-POINT EXPECTATION SYNDROME 80
- NORMALITY IS A RANGE 82
- WHY THE VARIATION? 84
- IS ULTRASOUND MORE ACCURATE? 85
- DATING APPROACHES AND INDIVIDUALISED CARE 88
- THE DUE DATE IS AN INTERVENTION 89

5. INDUCTION IN LATE PREGNANCY – YOUR BABY ISN'T LIKE A PUMPKIN 91

- A TINY BIT MORE HISTORY 91
- WHY IT'S COMPLICATED 94
- THE ACTUAL RISK OF STILLBIRTH 95
- BUT DOES INDUCTION MAKE A DIFFERENCE? 99
- WHAT'S NOT COMPARED, AND WHO'S NOT INCLUDED? 102
- BUT WHAT ABOUT THE ARRIVE TRIAL? 104
- DOES INDUCTION DECREASE THE CHANCE OF CAESAREAN? 107
- HOW HUMAN DECISIONS AFFECT RESEARCH FINDINGS 108

6. DOES MY BABY LOOK BIG IN THIS? 113

- WHAT'S THE PROBLEM? 114
- DEFINING BIG BABIES 115
- CENTILES, AVERAGES AND NORMALITY 116

THE ASSUMPTIONS AND THE EVIDENCE	117
ESTIMATING THE BABY'S WEIGHT	118
IS INDUCTION FOR SUSPECTED BIG BABIES BENEFICIAL?	119
DOWNSIDES OF INDUCING FOR SUSPECTED BIG BABIES	122
THE DOWNSIDES OF SCREENING	122
THE RECOMMENDATIONS AND THE REALITY	124
THE ROADS LESS TRAVELLED	125

7. TOO OLD, TOO FAT, TOO BLACK, TOO RISKY? 129

THE 'AT RISK' PROBLEM	130
THE DOWNSIDES OF LOOKING AT SINGLE FACTORS	132
OLDER WOMEN, INDUCTION AND RISK	135
MATERNAL AGE: THE WIDER ISSUES	139
UNDERSTANDING THE IMPORTANCE OF DISADVANTAGE	140
WHAT ABOUT LARGER WOMEN?	141
INDUCTION OUTCOMES IN LARGER WOMEN	143
TAKING A WOMAN-CENTRED VIEW	144
BMI AND SIZE: OTHER CONSIDERATIONS	146
MATERNAL RACE, RACISM AND INDUCTION	149
ANCESTRAL VARIATION AND WEATHERING	151
ROUTINE INDUCTION ISN'T THE ANSWER	153

8. ADDRESSING THE INDUCTION EPIDEMIC 155

SOLUTIONS THAT AREN'T HELPING	156
WHAT'S THE ANSWER?	158
BUT HOW?	159
REFRAMING NORMALITY, UNDERSTANDING RISK	162
LIVING IN OUR OWN TIME	163

REFERENCES 167

Foreword

In the past five decades, throughout high income countries and, more often in other parts of the world, we have seen a monumental shift towards an increasingly medicalised approach to pregnancy, labour and birth. In the UK this hastened dramatically with the publication of the Peel report[1] (1970) which, based on no reliable evidence, recommended 100% hospital birth, followed by a few days' postnatal stay; an objective justified on the grounds of "*The greater safety of hospital confinement...*" The word 'confinement' presenting an ironic paradox given that 1970 was also the year in which Germaine Greer published her landmark feminist text *The Female Eunuch*[2] and the Women's Liberation Movement was fast gaining momentum as part of second wave feminism.

Technical advances also played their part in facilitating the medicalisation of pregnancy and birth: Ultrasound scans gave us a 'window into the womb.' Manufactured prostaglandin and oxytocin enabled induction and the 'active management' of labour. Epidural analgesia enabled women to cope with the increased pain associated with induction and active management. And cardiotocography enabled clinicians to observe the fetal distress which too often resulted from the increased strength and frequency of augmented uterine contractions, so that obstetricians could then rescue the baby with an instrumental delivery or emergency caesarean section. Now I accept this is somewhat simplistic, and I am aware that some may consider this summary disrespectful, not least because for many well-meaning individuals, medicalised birth is advocated in the genuine belief that medical care equals safe care. Of course, obstetric intervention is sometimes necessary, and it can be life-saving for mothers and babies. But as a midwife who, throughout my 36 years of practice has also witnessed first-hand, the many negative consequences of these technocratic changes, who has seen the home birth rate fall ten-fold and the caesarean section rate increase almost ten-fold, with no proportional improvement in maternal and perinatal mortality and morbidity, and, perhaps most importantly, who has observed the erosion of women's confidence in their own ability to grow, birth and nurture their babies, concurrent with a dramatic rise in crippling anxiety, fear and birth trauma, it seems blindingly obvious that we are going in the wrong direction.

So why does all this matter, and, in particular, why does it matter right now? It matters because in the UK (and many other countries) we stand on the threshold of another significant shift in the way in which the pregnancy continuum is viewed and managed; we are about to take another step in the direction of technocratic birth. This is because the publication of the latest NICE *Inducing labour guideline*[3] includes several subtle, but potentially impactful changes compared to its 2008 predecessor.[4] These changes include (without good evidence) the offer of membrane sweeps for all women from 39 weeks (previously from 40 weeks for nulliparous women and from 41 weeks for parous women) and discussion of the risks of pregnancy progressing beyond 41 weeks (previously 42 weeks). The updated guideline also advocates that in early pregnancy we start discussing the possibility of induction of labour, at a time when it is certainly not needed, and indeed may never be needed, but will effectively begin that steady process of undermining women's (and clinicians') confidence in the body's amazing ability to labour and birth, if only normal physiology can be given a chance.

Induction of labour is important. It is important because it so often heralds the start of a relentless cascade of medical intervention. The start of a factory conveyor-belt model of labour and birth that is impersonal and dehumanising and strips women and their partners of choice and control. And if we do not take stock now, and ask some serious questions of our understanding of the physiological, psychological, social, spiritual and cultural aspects of the initiation and subsequent progress of labour and birth, an increasing proportion of pregnancies will be viewed as 'high risk' and normal physiological labour and birth will increasingly be condemned to historic oblivion.

This is why this latest book by Sara Wickham is so very timely and so very necessary. It is a counter-balance to so-called evidence-based guidelines, the recommendations of which, when scrutinised, are too often based on the 'knowledge and experience' of those who write them. As you read this book (if you don't know already) you will realise that Sara can 'think outside of the box' in such a way that few others can. Sara asks questions that others haven't considered and she isn't afraid to challenge our perceptions and to ask us not to take things for granted and accept the perceived norm, without careful and thoughtful analysis of the rationale and, crucially, the evidence. Sara also has the rare ability, not only to process complex research-based evidence and data herself, but to translate and explain them in such a way that they become easily understandable and make complete sense, even to the least research-minded among us. The amount of reliable, useful and powerful information in this book is, quite simply, staggering! It is a feminist text that recognises and respects women's rights and places the elements of choice and control exactly where they belong - in the hands of women themselves.

This book is essential reading (a rather clichéd and over-used phrase, but a truism here) for anyone involved with pregnancy, labour and birth. It is a book for policy makers, clinicians, maternity service managers, educators, birth workers and supporters. Most importantly, it is a book for all those who embark on the journey of pregnancy and who wish to make the best possible, well-informed decisions and choices that are right for them, right for their babies and right for their families.

Read, reflect on and relish the vast body of information contained within these pages. And, in whatever capacity you can, use it to question and challenge our relentless march toward induction of labour and medicalised labour and birth;

because the evidence suggests that only a minority may actually need it.

Julie Frohlich, November 2021

1. Ministry of Health (1970) Domiciliary Midwifery and Maternity Bed Needs: the Report of the Standing Maternity and Midwifery Advisory Committee (Sub-committee Chairman J. Peel), HMSO, London.
2. Greer G (1970) The Female Eunuch.
3. NICE (2021) Inducing labour guideline.
4. NICE (2008) Inducing labour guideline.

Introduction

I once met a woman who changed her Facebook picture when she got near her estimated due date. The new picture was of a roaring lion, and she had added some text. It said, *"No, I haven't f – g had it yet. I'll tell you when I have."*

She had, as you may have guessed, become exasperated with the number of enquiries that she was receiving as her pregnancy neared, reached and then passed the magical estimated due date, on which only one in twenty babies are actually born. If you've given birth in the past decade or two, you might be nodding in understanding. If you're pregnant right now, you might even be experiencing an urge to go and change your own cover photo. If so, go right ahead. No rush. There's plenty of time and I'll still be here when you get back. In fact, 'no rush' is a phrase that we could probably all do with hearing a bit more in our culture. But we'll get to that.

The Facebook picture was funny. It showed beautifully how one woman could stand up for what she needed. Yet it was also a sad indictment of our culture. Why should women have to do such things in order to get the peace they need at the end of pregnancy? I know women and families who have turned off their phones, unplugged from social media and posted signs on the front door; completely disconnecting from loved ones and those around them because of unwanted pressure about whether their baby has been born.

This isn't just about family and friends, though. Every day, I hear from women and families who are feeling unwanted pressure from medical professionals or concerned others who feel that their baby 'should have' been born by now, and who are offering or recommending intervention in order to make that happen. The recommendation for earlier and earlier induction of labour is becoming embedded in maternity care guidelines around the world. Many women are being offered other interventions such as membrane sweeping (where a midwife or doctor does an internal or vaginal examination in late pregnancy to try to stimulate labour) in the hope of avoiding 'full-blown' induction. Some people and documents try to suggest that this is not part of inducing labour. Many people don't agree. Induction is induction, and membrane sweeping is just as much an interference in the normal course of events as other mechanical or pharmaceutical methods of trying to bring on labour before the baby and the woman's body initiate this themselves. But whatever you think about that issue, the messages that we're sending by offering such procedures are the same. *Hurry up, hurry up; you're taking too long. It's not safe for the baby to stay in the womb.*

The fact is that, as a society, we have become impatient and fearful. We find it difficult to tolerate the uncertainty of not knowing exactly when something will happen. This doesn't just happen in relation to the end of pregnancy. The same trend can be seen in many other aspects of life as well. It's a source of immense stress for many people.

Until recently, most of the women who were told they needed induction were those whose had a medical condition or whose pregnancy was nearing 42 weeks, which western medicine has considered to be the upper end of 'term' for a few decades. Term has long been considered to be from 37 to 42 completed weeks of pregnancy. Some women have longer pregnancies than this. But the range of what is considered normal is narrowing. Many women are now offered induction even before they reach 40 weeks of pregnancy because their baby is deemed to be 'at risk' or 'high risk.'

In 2021, a panel who were drafting a new UK guideline (NICE 2021a) proposed offering induction at 39 weeks to older women, women with a higher BMI and women who conceived by IVF or other assisted reproductive technologies. The draft version of their guideline also suggested that clinicians consider offering induction at 39 weeks to Black, Brown, Asian and mixed-race women with uncomplicated pregnancies. These suggestions were met with a lot of concern. We clearly need to address the higher mortality rates in some groups of women, but there's no evidence to suggest that induction is the answer. This specific recommendation did not make the final guideline (NICE 2021b), but some of these women were already being offered earlier induction of labour before the new draft, and this is likely to continue. They need good information on which to base their decisions.

Increasingly, the 'at risk' group also includes women who are told that their baby is larger than average. This news can come as quite a nasty surprise. One day you think everything is lovely and normal, and then the next day a scan predicts that you have a big baby. Even though it is well known that ultrasound scans have a wide margin of error, especially in later pregnancy, women suddenly find that they are being given a date for induction. Many find this distressing, and they experience worry and angst, just when they should be resting and preparing for labour and birth.

These sweeping recommendations reflect just one, very narrow way of thinking. This is very problematic for many women and families, as well as for a lot of the people who work in systems of health care and who are worried about what's happening. A number of clinicians and managers are deeply concerned that maternity services do not have the capacity to handle as many inductions as are now happening, many of which are unnecessary. When services are overstretched, care can suffer and things can go wrong.

One of the key issues with the current situation is that medical organisations and systems of health care take a 'one size fits all' approach. Guidelines are based on population-level data, which don't account for individuality. This means that everyone who fits a certain criterion is offered the same thing. If you're over 35, you get offered induction at the same point as everyone else who is over 35. Never mind that there is huge variation in women who are over 35. Never mind that there isn't good evidence that early induction of labour would make a difference even if everyone had one.

In reality, bodies, babies and pregnancy lengths vary. In reality, we exhibit individual variation, and there is actually a wide span of time in which babies can be born and be healthy.

In other words, as I will discuss in this book, normal is a range and not just one fixed point. One size hardly ever fits all!

Of course, induction can and often does make a huge difference if a woman or baby has a medical condition. I'll reiterate that throughout this book. Induction of labour is absolutely the right decision for some women and families. There are some conditions that can only be resolved by the baby being born. I'm not anti-induction. I'm anti using limited and cherry-picked evidence and deceptive claims about risk to try to persuade entire groups of women to hand over control of their bodies and undergo intervention in the name of safety, when the recommendations aren't based on good science or an understanding of the wider consequences of such actions and may cause harm.

But induction is increasingly being offered to women who don't have medical conditions. As a result, the induction rate is rising, especially in high-income countries, and the effects are worrying. Induction of labour is a multi-stage medical intervention involving invasive procedures and/or drugs. And medical interventions, procedures and drugs carry risks as well as potential benefits.

As a midwife who has attended hundreds of births and a researcher who has researched induction of labour for more than twenty-five years, I am really concerned about what is happening. Our culture has rapidly embraced a medical approach to pregnancy and birth which isn't based on sound evidence or clear thinking. This approach fails to consider the individual, focuses on short-term, physical outcomes and ignores medium- and long-term health and the psychological and social consequences of induction. The guidelines that underpin the medical approach (e.g. NICE 2021b) consider only a small proportion of the research that has been carried out in this area. They don't acknowledge that some of the studies are flawed and limited in what they can tell us. They don't include the valuable knowledge that we can gain from experts in disciplines like psychology, anthropology, history and sociology. They haven't included the papers in which people have raised concerns about the value of routine induction. They don't consider the views and experiences of women and families. It sometimes seems as if evidence is cherry picked to underpin arguments for routine induction, regardless of whether or not that evidence is robust.

People need the bigger picture. It's time we had a book exploring the benefits of going into labour in your own time, and explaining the downsides to interfering without good cause. We need a book that discusses variation and individual differences and explains why the idea of a fixed due date that is calculated the same way for everybody is nonsensical. A book rooted in the idea that the female body knows how to grow, birth and feed babies, and not in the medical myth that our bodies are risky, unstable and untrustworthy, or that women's knowledge and pain is less valid than men's. We need more books that strip back the myths, unpack the evidence, tell women's stories and show that, in some cases, the emperor is actually naked.

So here is that book. I've written it for anyone questioning the value of routine induction or concerned about rising induction rates. It's for those who wonder whether we should be interfering so much at the end of pregnancy, or who want to explore other ways of thinking about this.

This book is probably not for anyone who is very committed to induction or has already decided to have their labour induced (unless you're questioning that and want a different perspective). I'm not going to explain what induction entails or look at the pros and cons in detail. I've already written a popular book discussing those things: 'Inducing Labour: making informed decisions' (Wickham 2018a). I hope people will find this one just as useful.

I begin this book by focusing on what's normal, and on the value of spontaneous labour. I'll go on to answer the million pound question: why doesn't every woman get to birth in her own way? That is, how have we got to where we are? It's vital to understand that. We can't begin to unpick the current situation until we understand how it came about, and what we need to challenge in order to overcome it. Chapter three looks at the changing guidance and shares the views and voices of women, including some of those who care for other women. This is a neglected area, and it needs our focus.

I'm then going to look at several of the specific issues that I've already mentioned in this introduction. There's a chapter on due dates, timing and why it's so important to look at women as individuals. I'm going to explain (in a really friendly way – no mathematical knowledge required!) what the obstetric research does and does not tell us about induction in very late pregnancy. There's a chapter on the issues and research relating to suspected big babies, and another looking at whether certain groups of women really are at higher risk. I have shared (with permission, of course) the words of many women and caregivers, and you will see these throughout the book with pseudonyms chosen by those who have shared their experiences with me for the book.

If you read this book like a novel, you'll notice that I cross reference and repeat myself a bit. That's because some people will be desperate for the information in one section and they'll head straight there. Thank you for being patient with that.

At this point in history, maternity care isn't serving women, babies and families well. Moves to advise more and more women to have an induction of labour are a reflection of this. It's my hope that this book will help to change that. It's not okay that women are having to turn off their phones at the end of pregnancy, or post pictures asking people to stop hassling them. We need to change our approach to one that supports women and babies, respects physiology, is based on evidence and takes wider outcomes into account. We need individualised care. Unless there is a genuine medical condition where the benefits of intervention outweigh the downsides (and it is, of course, still the woman who gets to make that decision), there's no reason to try to hurry things up and prevent women from giving birth in their own time.

Sara Wickham. Wiltshire, England. November 2021.

1. The advantages of the waiting days

As Ruth rocked her hips while giving a few gentle, nudgy pushes, I looked up at the moon. It was full and round through the patio doors, left open in the hope of clearing the July heat which had built up in the birth centre. It's not usually helpful to watch birthing women. Now and again they want focused eye contact with someone they trust, but most often that's their partner. Sometimes even their gaze is too much. On the whole, the flow of oxytocin and other birth hormones and thus the journey of labour itself tends to work best when unobserved. So as a midwife I try to find something else to give my focus to. Or at least I pretend to be fully focused on the something else, while in reality I'm keeping a check on things out of the corner of my eye. Sometimes I knit. But it was too hot for that. On that night, I was seemingly admiring the purples of the summer night sky.

James' eyes had widened when he saw the full moon emerge from behind the trees that shielded the birth centre's garden from public view, and we had shared a smile. Ruth had been convinced for weeks that she would go into labour at the full moon, and she had been right. As a scientist, James thought it was coincidence, and the pair had teased each other about it until Ruth needed to focus on the sensations of labour. Now, it would likely become a part of story they told about their birth. *"Our baby decided to be born on the full moon."*

I watched James pull his phone from his pocket, wanting to capture the moment. I didn't have the heart to tell him that, like many dads-to-be before him, he would find it became just a pinprick on the screen. It's always lovely to see the moon at a birth, but she doesn't like to take centre stage in the photos.

Not that I want to paint an overly romantic picture of birth. The moon *was* lovely that night, but two flies were noisily trying for a baby of their own near the lamp, and my tee shirt sported a small jammy handprint which I hadn't yet found time to sponge off. I was also having a debate in my head about whether I had time to nip out quickly. If I had to bet on it, I would have predicted that birth was about half an hour away. But I had been a midwife for a decade by then. I knew better than to put money on that kind of thing. Because babies come in their own time. No matter what the moon is doing. Women's bodies work to their own rhythms, too. And, as a midwife, the best and safest thing I can do at a birth is to watch, wait, be vigilant lest my help be needed, but otherwise allow things to unfold. It's almost always better that way.

In this chapter, I'll explain why that's also usually the case when it comes to awaiting the onset of labour.

The value of ripening

"In the last weeks of pregnancy, maternal antibodies are passed to the baby - antibodies that will help fight infections in the first days and weeks of life. The baby gains weight and strength, stores iron, and develops more coordinated sucking and swallowing abilities. His lungs mature, and he stores brown fat that will help him maintain body temperature in the first days and weeks following birth. The maturing baby and the aging placenta trigger a prostaglandin increase that softens the cervix in readiness for effacement and dilatation. A rise in estrogen and a decrease in progesterone increase the uterine sensitivity to oxytocin. The baby moves down into the pelvis. Contractions in the last weeks may start the effacement and dilation of the cervix. A burst of energy helps pregnant women make final preparations, and insomnia prepares them for the start of round-the-clock parenting.

"The watchful waiting and the intense wanting of the big day to arrive are all part of nature's plan. When the baby, uterus, placenta, and hormones are ready, labor will start. Additionally, all that preparation sets the stage for an easier labor and a fully mature baby who is physiologically stable and able to breastfeed well right from the start." (Lothian 2006: 43).

Since Judith Lothian (2006) wrote those two paragraphs, which I often read aloud when talking to women and families about the benefits of waiting for labour to start on its own, many studies showing other benefits to awaiting spontaneous labour have been published. We'll look at those throughout this chapter. But I've never found a more succinct description than Lothian's of the many aspects of health and birth that are optimised when we let the baby decide when labour starts.

As far as we know at this point in history, it is the baby who decides when to be born. If we let things be, that is. But we don't know for sure what happens. Early researchers theorised that the onset of labour was affected by the release of cortisol from the baby, which stimulates the mother to produce hormones (Gennser *et al* 1977). Later, a study on birthing mice (yes, really!) suggested that labour is initiated when the baby's lungs are fully mature. Condon *et al* (2004) demonstrated that, when the fetal lungs are completely ready for life in air, they make a type of protein which sends a wave of prostaglandins through the mother's body. Prostaglandins are hormones that play a key part in starting labour. They are also used in some induction drugs, but I'm not going to focus on that here.

Despite having some theories, we still don't know exactly what makes labour start. It may be a combination of several things working together. We are confident that the baby's physiology plays a significant part. This fact alone should surely make us pause before trying to start labour by artificial means. If labour hasn't started yet, then it may be because the baby's lungs or other body systems aren't yet fully ready for life in air. But that's merely the first advantage to waiting. There are many more.

The hormonal orchestra

As one reviewer summarised, *"The most compelling reason to let labor begin on its own may be to allow the birth hormones to regulate labor and birth, breastfeeding, and attachment as nature intends."* (Amis 2014: 179).

Since Hippocrates embedded the guiding principle of *primum non nocere*, or *'first, do no harm'* into health care, doctors and other practitioners have been urged to interfere only when the benefits of intervention outweigh the risks. This is particularly important when it comes to pregnancy and birth. For a start, pregnancy and birth are not disease processes. And, as there is so much that we still don't understand about them, we would do well to respect the physiological process unless there's truly a good reason not to. Medical intervention is only occasionally truly warranted because, on the whole, birth already works really well.

"The idiom 'if it ain't broke, don't fix it' may not be the most erudite of phrases, but it effectively contains the maxim that not only is it pointless to try to improve upon a system that already works well; the interference itself may be harmful and/or lead to unwanted knock-on effects or further harms." (Wickham & Robinson 2010).

This is further illustrated by a wonderful article by midwife Tricia Anderson, who wrote about what would happen if we took cats into a laboratory to give birth, by means of illustrating the harm that can come from disturbing the hormonal dance of labour.

"In the laboratory, the labouring cats could hear the sound of other cats in distress, and there were no private dark corners for them to retreat to, but only rows of brightly-lit cages under constant scrutiny of the scientists. And the scientists studied the labouring cats in their brightly-lit cages for many years, and saw that their labours were erratic, how they slowed down and even stopped, and how heartbreakingly distressed the cats were. Their mews and their cries were terrible. They saw how many of the kittens were deprived of oxygen and were born shocked and needing resuscitation. And, after many years the scientists concluded 'well, it seems that cats do not labour very well'." (Anderson 2002: 65).

A similar thing has happened to human women. Labour and birth have now been routinely managed for decades, and this management has included convincing people that the female body isn't terribly good at pregnancy and birth. Yet, like the cats in the story above, a good part of the problem that we see today is the interference itself. If we kept the aspects of western medicine that can truly be shown to be effective –

like good hygiene, and antibiotics, blood transfusion and surgery in (and only in) cases when they are truly warranted – then how would things be different? Just as importantly, what are we losing through routine interference?

Thanks to Australian General Practitioner Sarah Buckley, we can now answer that. She compiled an extensive summary of the research into the hormones that are involved in regulating labour and birth. Her work considered the possible impacts of scheduled birth (by which we mean inducing labour or performing a caesarean section before labour begins spontaneously). For a start, some women can experience less efficient contractions, although they may feel very painful. Having less efficient contractions can mean that efforts to induce labour don't work, which can in turn lead to more interventions such as instrumental birth (forceps or vacuum) or a caesarean. It can also lead to more bleeding. All of these things can have later effects as well and influence what happens in future births as well as the options that might be open to the woman. Scheduled birth can also negatively affect breast feeding, bonding with the baby and how the woman's body adapts during and after birth (Buckley 2015: xii).

Buckley (2015) found that scheduled birth can have negative effects on babies too. The processes that protect them after birth may be immature if labour is induced (or if they are born by scheduled caesarean). This can include some of the hormonal processes that work during labour, which means that babies may be more likely to become distressed if labour is induced, as they weren't ready to be born. They have a greater chance of having breathing difficulties after birth (again, because they may not have been ready to be born) and difficulties with regulating their blood sugar and their body temperature. Their brain, hormone and other organ systems may not be fully mature and there may also be effects that we do not fully understand (Buckley 2015: xii).

Allowing labour to begin spontaneously ensures that the hormones of pregnancy and birth, which have now been shown to have myriad and far-reaching beneficial effects, have the best possible chance of working as nature intended. Since the research into this area is relatively new, it is likely that we have only begun to scratch the surface of our understanding about the effects of these hormones on women's and babies' future health. But our knowledge is growing, and each new study seems to confirm this further. Midwifery Professor Hannah Dahlen *et al* (2013) suggested that events during the intrapartum (or 'in labour') period, including the synthetic oxytocin used in induction of labour, can *"...affect the ... subsequent health of the mother and offspring."* Dahlen (2015) later noted that being born as nature intended, *"...is good for you."* Many body systems are affected by the hormones of birth, and all can be negatively impacted by unnecessary interference.

Avoiding the problems of being born too early

One really important benefit to awaiting spontaneous labour is that it guarantees that the baby won't be born too early as the result of inducing labour. This situation happens more often than you might think, for instance because of an incorrect due date or ultrasound error. Unless pregnancy was conceived outside the womb or sex only happened once, we cannot be sure of a baby's gestational age, or how many weeks pregnant a woman was when her baby was born. Even then, babies develop at different rates. Some might be ready to initiate labour at 36 weeks of pregnancy, and some might wait beyond 42. As I will discuss in chapter four, due dates are only guesses, no matter how they are calculated.

So when we induce labour (or do an elective caesarean before labour starts), there is always a chance that we will be causing the baby to be born sooner than is ideal. With some countries' obstetric guidelines now recommending that induction should be offered at or around 39 weeks of pregnancy, this chance increases. So awaiting spontaneous labour means we avoid the problem of iatrogenic (or medically caused) prematurity and all the potential difficulties this might cause the baby, which I discuss below.

Researchers now know quite a bit about the risks that arise from being born too early. In fact, we have changed the way we discuss gestational age as a result of this knowledge. For a long time, we talked about preterm babies (those born before 37 completed weeks of pregnancy), term babies (37-42 completed weeks) and post-term babies, which were the babies born after 42 completed weeks. But researchers and health professionals have expanded their definitions of time frames over the past few years. That's because we now understand that gestational age, *"…represents a continuum in which risk and severity of adverse outcomes increase with decreasing gestational age, but where measurable effects can be detected even very close to full term."* (Gill & Boyle 2017: 194).

In other words, there are detectable differences between babies born at 37 or 38 weeks of pregnancy and babies born at 41 weeks of pregnancy. These differences tend to reflect the benefits that come from staying in the womb as long as is needed for that particular baby to develop fully mature organs and systems. Yes, there are plenty of babies who were born after their mums went into labour at 37 or 38 weeks who are fine. But, because babies initiate labour themselves, it's possible that those particular babies were ready to be born then, but that others of the same age might not be. You won't necessarily see the differences by comparing two or more specific babies either. We're all unique. Unborn babies develop at different rates, just as older babies, toddlers and teenagers develop at different rates. But we can see some differences on a population basis, by which I mean when we compare the health of large numbers of babies born at various gestational ages.

So researchers and health professionals now talk about 'late preterm' babies (those born between 34 and 36 completed weeks of pregnancy) and 'early term' babies (those born in gestational weeks 37 and 38). Babies born in weeks 39, 40 and 41 are described as full term and babies born from 42 weeks are described as post-term. There are also several other categories for babies born preterm, but I won't go into those here, as they're not relevant to what we're discussing.

It is well understood that babies born preterm are at higher risk of many health conditions. But even babies who are born in the late preterm and early term periods are at increased risk of having a number of adverse outcomes compared with babies born at full term. These include breathing difficulties, infection, hypoglycaemia (or low blood sugar), difficulty regulating their temperature, jaundice and feeding difficulties (Loftin *et al* 2010, Brown *et al* 2014, Boyle *et al* 2015, Gill & Boyle 2017).

For the most part, these problems aren't serious, but they can result in prolonged hospitalisation (Gill & Boyle 2017). Children born before full term (39-41 weeks gestation) are also at increased risk of adverse cognitive (or learning related) outcomes (Noble *et al* 2012, Chan *et al* 2016). We also know that brain volume increases when babies are allowed to stay in the womb for longer (El Marroun *et al* 2020). A paper from The Millenium Cohort Study showed that, *"...children born at earlier gestational ages are more likely to experience SEN* [special educational needs], *have more complex SEN and require support in multiple facets of learning."* (Alterman *et al* 2021). Baby girls born in the late preterm and early term period have more emotional challenges at 36 months of age compared to those born at term (Stene-Larsen *et al* 2016). The academic and cognitive benefits that come from being born later may be even higher in families who are disadvantaged (Figlio *et al* 2016). These are just a few of the studies to illustrate the key points. Many more show the same things.

Babies born before full term are also more likely to experience breast feeding issues (Lutsiv *et al* 2013, Goyal *et al* 2014). One large study found that the rate of breast feeding problems decreases with each week of gestational age. In other words, the later a baby is born, the less likely it will be to have breast feeding problems (Lutsiv *et al* 2013). As Gill and Boyle (2017) note, *"Decreased likelihood of breast feeding may be important with respect to later outcomes, given the known long-term health and neurodevelopmental benefits of breast milk."*

Again, this does not mean that every baby born preterm will be negatively affected. We often don't know (because researchers don't always look at this) whether the babies in these studies were born after a spontaneous or induced labour. This is a real oversight, because it could be crucial to know whether the babies who determine their own time of birth are less likely to have difficulty if born at a particular gestational age than those whose mums' labour was induced. Researchers have called for more data to be collected on iatrogenic prematurity for some time now (Fuchs & Wapner 2006). Sadly, the organisations promoting induction don't seem interested in acknowledging that a major benefit of spontaneous labour, and thus a major downside of induction and scheduled or elective caesarean, is that it means many babies are now born before they are ready.

Another sad fact is that some data have shown that a baby who is born in the late preterm period is three times more likely to die in the first year of their life than a baby who was born at full term (Mathews & MacDorman 2013). We urgently need more data on this, and to know whether this is more likely if birth happens before the baby is ready, because of induction or elective caesarean, whatever the underlying cause(s), but it is not being adequately researched. One reason we need more data is that the main reason given for preventing some women from experiencing spontaneous labour is that they have a slightly higher chance of having a stillborn baby. If induction is leading to a higher chance of death in the first year of life (a time frame in which mortality is not usually measured in induction studies) then it may be that induction is simply delaying the death of some babies. Or it could be that induction prevents the death of some of the babies who might have been stillborn without it, while at the same time leading to the deaths of others, because it means that they are born before they were ready, and their health suffers as a result.

It is imperative that we take a longer view on the consequences of interfering with labour and birth. Otherwise, we are not giving full and accurate information to women and families. All of these physical, mental, emotional, cognitive and developmental consequences have an impact on all of us, because they can affect people's wellbeing and needs for the rest of their life.

The problem of being born too early is not going away anytime soon. We can never be certain that we have calculated a baby's gestational age correctly; it is always an *estimated* due date. As I have explained, inducing labour (and thus overriding the baby's decision about when to be born) means that there is always a chance that we will be causing a baby to be born before it is ready. If there is a serious issue with the mother's and/or baby's health, causing the baby to be born early may well be justifiable. Conditions such as pre-eclampsia in the mother, for instance, can become serious very quickly and this is a very good reason to induce labour. There are also some babies who are truly at risk (for instance because of blood-related disorders) and who need to be born early so they can be given life-saving treatment. But most inductions nowadays are not done for these reasons. So questions should always be asked about whether the benefits of induction truly outweigh the risks of overriding the benefits of allowing labour to begin spontaneously, and at a time dictated by the baby's and mother's physiology.

This risk of being born too early doesn't go away even when a woman is thought to be 41 or more weeks pregnant, although the chance of a premature baby is less then. But the risk of being born too early is of particular concern when induction is recommended at 39 weeks. As I will discuss in chapter four, the margin of error in estimating the due date can be quite wide, and there is considerable variation between individuals. So a key advantage to awaiting spontaneous labour is that there is far less chance of the baby having any of the conditions or complications that can arise from having been made to be born before it is ready.

Other benefits of spontaneous labour for babies

I have already discussed how waiting for spontaneous labour is advantageous for the baby because it avoids the risks of being born in the preterm or early term period. I noted some of the risks of scheduled birth as they relate to the hormonal regulation of birth. There are other advantages to spontaneous labour for the baby too. Many of these centre around the fact that a baby whose labour has begun spontaneously is less likely to be subjected to drugs, procedures and interventions which each carry risks and may lead to further interventions.

Babies born after labour starts spontaneously are more likely to have a straightforward, physiological birth. They are less likely to be born by forceps and caesarean, which both carry risks. Yes, there is some debate about this, because some very medicalised studies say otherwise. I will discuss this more fully in later chapters. Suffice to say, if you look at real-life data and consider the wider picture of how the studies were carried out, there's good evidence that induction increases the chance of caesarean. Babies born after a spontaneous onset of labour are less likely to need special or intensive care. If they are born in hospital, they are more likely to go home sooner after spontaneous labour, although this can depend on whether the induction was for a medical reason or just because the woman and/or baby was perceived to be at higher risk. There have been numerous studies, books and reviews which have consistently found and shared the same outcomes for many years (Inch 1982, Lothian 2006, Baud *et al* 2013, Amis 2014, Buckley 2015, Reed 2018, Wickham 2018a, Rydahl *et al* 2019, Seijmonsbergen-Schermers *et al* 2020, Dahlen *et al* 2021, Levine *et al* 2021).

The study by Dahlen *et al* (2021) is one of the most recent and also one of the most comprehensive. It was ground-breaking in that the researchers, *"…compared intrapartum interventions and outcomes for mothers, neonates and children up to 16 years, for induction of labour (IOL) versus spontaneous labour onset in uncomplicated term pregnancies with live births."* (Dahlen *et al* 2021). This time span goes far beyond what any other group of researchers have considered, and the data set was very large, involving 474,652 births. Of those women, 69,397 (15%) had their labour induced for non-medical reasons. This shows just how common unwarranted induction is becoming, and many midwives and doctors say that the rate is rising.

Dahlen *et al*'s (2021) findings also showed that induction of labour leads to more intervention and more adverse maternal, neonatal and child outcomes.

"Between birth and 16 years of age, and controlled for year of birth, their children [born after induction] *had higher odds of birth asphyxia, birth trauma, respiratory disorders, major resuscitation at birth and hospitalisation for infection."* (Dahlen *et al* 2021).

The authors note that, in their research, *"…only hospital admissions were examined and hence more serious illnesses."* (Dahlen *et al* 2021). It's therefore possible that the chance of more minor illness might be increased as well, but we can't know that from this particular study. Worryingly, although the induction rate had tripled in some groups in the 16 years spanned by the study, Dahlen *et al* (2021) found that there had been no reduction in stillbirth. This is of huge concern, as possible reduction in the chance of stillbirth is the reason often given to support a recommendation of induction, especially when there are no medical indications for induction.

Advantages of spontaneous labour for women

In *Why Induction Matters*, midwife and author Rachel Reed (2018) shares the words of Mariana, who describes her experience of physiological labour.

"Feeling how my body communicated with me was unbelievable. The way I could work with my baby on his way out was so satisfying! Also I felt protected. I was in control of everything so the pain was perfectly manageable. The power I felt for doing this huge thing, giving birth, on my own, was unbelievable. I felt like super woman. I slept, I ate, I danced, I kissed. We were in our own time. Mariana." (Reed 2018: 91).

Most of what I've discussed so far has concerned the physical and physiological benefits to the baby of allowing labour to begin spontaneously, which means that women like Mariana and Ruth are more likely to experience physiological labour. Induction of labour researchers don't tend to measure whether women feel in control, protected or 'like super woman.' Those aren't common outcome measures in randomised controlled trials.

Outcome measures also tend not to include the amount of dancing or kissing that women engage in during labour. But the emotional and psychological benefits are just as important (and sometimes more so) to women and families as the physical benefits of spontaneous labour for women. They can help us to become strong parents. There's more on women's experiences in chapter three, and I will also look at the less tangible benefits of allowing labour to begin spontaneously in the next section. But I will note for the sake of completeness here that, when I have sought and searched for papers and experiences of spontaneous and induced labour for books and studies throughout my career, there's a definite trend. Yes, there are a few women who dislike spontaneous labour and prefer induction. But overall, there are far more accounts of women being happy with spontaneous labour and unhappy with their induction experience than the other way around.

There are numerous physical benefits for women to going into spontaneous labour. Many of these overlap with the benefits for babies that I have already mentioned. Women whose labour starts spontaneously are less likely to have interventions, including drugs, continuous electronic fetal monitoring, and intravenous drips. They are less likely to need pharmaceutical pain relief. They are likely to have fewer vaginal examinations. They have a lower chance of being told they need an instrumental birth or a caesarean section, which also means they have a lower chance of having one or more of the long-term complications of these. They are more likely to be able to give birth at a place of their choosing and, if they birth in hospital, they are likely to be able to go home sooner.

They are less likely to have a postpartum haemorrhage (PPH) and psychological trauma after their birth. For more on this, see Lothian (2006), Baud *et al* (2013), Buckley (2015), Reed (2018), Wickham (2018a), Rydahl *et al* (2019), Seijmonsbergen-Schermers *et al* (2020), Dahlen *et al* (2021).

I have already mentioned a recent and large study which looked at the long-term outcomes after induction (Dahlen *et al* 2021). This study also found that:

"Women with uncomplicated pregnancies who had their labour induced had higher rates of epidural/spinal analgesia, CS (except for multiparous women induced at between 37 and 40 weeks gestation), instrumental birth, episiotomy and PPH than women with a similar risk profile who went into labour spontaneously ... IOL for non-medical reasons was associated with higher birth interventions, particularly in primiparous women, and more adverse maternal, neonatal and child outcomes for most variables assessed." (Dahlen *et al* 2021).

I want to mention one more study, whose findings relate to this and the previous section. Seijmonsbergen-Schermers *et al* (2020) considered 'avoidable harm' in their research. They concluded that it is vital to study the long-term disadvantages of interfering with normal physiology and imposing induction-related interventions upon women's health.

"Inducing women to prevent small absolute risks based on trials undertaken with very discrete populations neglects these warnings. Besides, a small increase in absolute risk does not necessarily mean that outcomes will be improved if labor is induced. Without the full picture of longer term outcomes from single and multiple cumulative interventions, and in the absence of a clear understanding of the compiled morbidity that may eventuate over a woman's life time of reproduction, it is not possible to achieve fully informed judgements." Seijmonsbergen-Schermers *et al* (2020).

It's clear that the benefits of spontaneous labour for women are significant and far-reaching. And inducing labour may negatively affect a woman for the rest of her life. Intervention also carries many knock-on effects which are not beneficial to women. This is particularly true when oxytocin is given by intravenous drip, as this can have many unwanted and harmful effects on women and babies (Buckley 2015). For all the reasons discussed in this chapter, as Seijmonsbergen-Schermers *et al* (2020) explain, we have to ask whether induction is justified when a small increase in absolute risk in one area is offset against the many other harms that induction can lead to for both mother and baby.

Again, if there is a genuine medical condition, the benefit may well outweigh the risk. That isn't in question. The issue is that routine induction is nowadays offered simply because of a possible slight increase in the risk of immediate neonatal mortality (stillbirth), which we now know may be offset by a greater chance of mortality in the longer term.

Another issue is that, while we have some good data, many aspects of women's experiences aren't considered here. I will look at these in chapter three, but I want to end this chapter by discussing just one wider benefit of spontaneous labour. This is not generally considered or researched, but it's something that many of us are beginning to think about. Partly because we've come to realise that our fast-paced, screen-focused, urgency-filled and disconnected way of life isn't always providing what we need and it may not sustain the parts of us that scientific research tends not to reach.

Wider benefits, nesting and the time of zwischen

"She's curled up on the couch, waiting, a ball of baby and emotions. A scrambled pile of books on pregnancy, labor, baby names, breastfeeding; not one more word can be absorbed. The birth supplies are loaded in a laundry basket, ready for action. The freezer is filled with meals, the car seat installed, the camera charged. It's time to hurry up and wait. Not a comfortable place to be, but wholly necessary. The last days of pregnancy - sometimes stretching to agonizing weeks - are a distinct place, time, event, stage. It is a time of in between. Neither here nor there. Your old self and your new self, balanced on the edge of a pregnancy. One foot in your old world, one foot in a new world." (Studelska 2012).

Midwife Jana Studelska (2012) discusses how she uses the German word zwischen (meaning between) to describe the in-between time in very late pregnancy when we are waiting for labour to start. This time doesn't have a name in English, but perhaps it should have. It's also not something that is often or openly discussed, but I have heard many women and midwives talk about there being a benefit to 'sitting with the waiting' in the days leading up to labour. I have also interviewed midwives from around the world about their approach to late pregnancy. Here's a quote from one of my research participants about her own experience:

"It gave me time to get my head around it all, especially as I couldn't leave work that early. It was hard, to deal with the uncertainty, but also sort of somehow, I suppose healing is the word that comes to mind. It gave me space to have weird dreams and then work through them. To face my fears, and talk myself down. Two of my friends came round and they cooked and put meals in the freezer for us for after he was born. So the practical things that you do to adjust in that space are one thing. But having time to adjust in ways I didn't even know I was adjusting ... can't put a price on that. Can't put a name to it either [laughs]. *But it was real."* (Kris).

There's absolutely no room for this sort of thing in the modern medical approach to the end of pregnancy, as I'll discuss in the next chapter. That's because the focus is all on the short-term physical aspects. Research funding isn't often given to experiences that are more psychologically, socially or spiritually focused.

But it's a very real thing for many women and families, and acknowledging it can offer tangible benefits. It's easy to understand that there are social and practical advantages to having some adjustment time at the end of pregnancy. The parents-to-be can spend time together, talking about the upcoming birth and sharing thoughts and feelings about becoming parents. It can be a time to fill the freezer and make a rota of friends who have offered to help with housework. Women often begin to 'nest' as labour nears, and this can mean anything from having an urge to make their space clean and tidy to embarking on a full-scale, whole house declutter. (Not joking about this. It was one of the few occasions where I abandoned my usual 'only you can decide what's right for you' mantra and gently suggested at the end of an antenatal visit that 41 and a half weeks of pregnancy might not be the best time to empty every cupboard in the kitchen, with a plan to declutter the whole house over the next couple of weeks. If you think that was too harsh, then I can live with that. The baby was born eighteen hours later, and its parents were very happy that I recommended doing one cupboard at a time).

The point is that many women and parents have found value in their experience of the last few days of pregnancy. This is especially the case where women are expected to work until 38 weeks of pregnancy, which is a recent phenomenon. They describe the benefits of having time to adjust, in whatever way they need to adjust. People adjust their house, the contents of their hospital bag, the fairy lights that they've hung around the birth pool, their headspace or their hopes and dreams. Maybe all of the above. There's also something in the idea of letting go of control; of being mindful, and letting the hormonal orchestra play. In our modern world, many parents are – quite understandably – desperate to meet their baby. Women can't wait to not be big and pregnant anymore, to move onto the next stage. That's perhaps one reason why induction appeals to some people. But I've heard enough women talk about what they gained in those last few days of pregnancy for me to feel it's worth writing about as a benefit of waiting. Maybe one day we will open our minds and look more closely at the less tangible benefits that some women attribute to awaiting spontaneous labour.

Summarising the benefits

In this chapter, I've discussed how awaiting spontaneous labour has significant and varied physical, physiological, psychological and other short-, medium- and long-term health and wider benefits for women, babies and families.

These benefits have been demonstrated by numerous studies carried out over several decades, and we know about even more from the lived experience of parents and professionals.

No study or review of studies on induction of labour has come anywhere near showing that offering induction on a routine basis would come even close to exceeding the many short-, medium- and long-term benefits to healthy women and babies of awaiting spontaneous labour. If a particular woman and/or baby has a condition that warrants earlier birth, then the benefits of induction of labour (or an elective caesarean) may well outweigh the benefits of spontaneous labour and the risks of intervention. But this decision needs to be made on an individual basis. It's also important to note that, if we take the evidence into account, such decisions should be made on the basis of there being actual pathology (or illness/ abnormality) rather than just a slightly increased chance of a problem. In later chapters, I will look further at what happens when induction or elective caesarean is offered simply for 'being at risk,' and why this is often questionable.

One of the most significant risks of routinely offering induction (especially when this is offered at or around 39 weeks) is that babies may be born too early. Equally worrying is the chance that any small theoretical reduction in stillbirth among certain groups is offset by an increase in infant mortality following induced labour. Both of these are serious and under-researched concerns which have been ignored by policy makers. But these concerns need to be taken into account when anyone, whether making guidelines or making decisions about their own body, is considering whether the benefits of inducing labour outweigh the benefits of awaiting the spontaneous, physiological onset of labour.

In the next chapter, I will look at how we have come to be in the current situation and ask how our society has ended up in a state where an intervention which has many downsides is offered routinely? Especially when so much evidence shows that waiting for spontaneous labour would be a better default option unless there is a genuine complication.

2. Why doesn't every woman get to birth in her own way?

"The majority of obstetricians, everywhere, have become so convinced that the natural process of birth is fraught with dangers which their increasingly sophisticated technological interventions are increasingly capable of minimizing. Amazingly, they have managed, without producing any valid supporting evidence, to persuade the majority of people, medical and lay, that they are right and the maternity service has been organized in accordance with this unjustifiable hypothesis." (Tew 1986: 671).

I'll never forget the look in George's eyes as he watched his first baby being born. He was behind his partner Eliza in the birth pool; holding her tenderly and kneeling up so that he could watch over her shoulder as their baby slipped from her body. It was just after midnight and their kitchen was lit by an assortment of fairy lights and table lamps. There was a sense of timelessness in the room, which still held the smell of the chicken soup and freshly baked bread that we had all shared just a couple of hours earlier.

George gazed in wonder at his baby boy as the tiny new person floated in the pool, seemingly not yet fully aware that he had even left the womb. Watching his wife give birth in her own time and in her own power was, George said later, the most amazing thing he had ever seen. He then showered Eliza with kisses, telling her how proud of her he was. Tears filled his eyes as he gently reached to stroke their little boy's head with one finger.

A few minutes later he looked up at me with a question.

"Why doesn't every woman get to birth in her own way?" he whispered. *"This is so different from what you see on the telly."*

The million pound questions

George wasn't the first person to ask me a question like that, and he won't be the last. Many of the people who have found their way to gentle, holistic, woman-centred, and midwifery-led approaches to birth wonder why everyone doesn't do the same. People ask a couple of related questions as well. The first is to wonder how we got to the situation we are in now, in which birth is routinely interfered with. Often, they have seen that this interference can do more harm than good. Then, they ask why, when we've got a growing mountain of evidence to suggest that the modern, medical approach to birth isn't working, isn't kind and isn't the best for all women and babies, we haven't changed our approach.

Here are the brief answers to each of those questions and a few others, as a kind of overview to what I'm going to discuss in this chapter. First, there are many reasons that most people don't have the kind of birth that Eliza and George experienced. Some don't know it's an option. Some don't have the resources to question, or to be able to act on their wishes and decisions. Many have been convinced that birth is dangerous and is much better done in hospital where doctors are at hand. Some of those who like the idea of a more woman-centred, individualised and holistic approach are talked out of it by well-meaning but fearful family, friends or caregivers. Medically managed hospital birth has become the norm, and many people don't like going against the norm.

That's entirely understandable. Humans have a tendency to assume that *'what is, must be best.'* (Porter & Macintyre 1984, van Teijlingen *et al* 2003). In other words, many people have long thought that those who run countries or maternity services must surely always be offering us the best possible service or care. So it doesn't occur to some people to question what's on offer, or to look for alternatives. But at the same time, there is a growing distrust in experts and professionals and we're living in an age in which there is a huge amount of information. Modern technologies allow for anyone to call themselves an expert, but there is no correlation between the number of followers someone has and the quality of the information they are sharing. It can be confusing and hard to know who and what to trust.

The short answer to the question about how we got to where we are today is that the approach taken to childbirth in many high-income countries nowadays is rooted in some historical ideas which started taking hold about three hundred years ago. These ideas have changed and influenced every facet of our culture and society. Like every innovation, idea or technology, they have brought advantages and disadvantages. In my view, it's worth trying to understand, because this is at the very heart of the situation we face.

I've already partly answered the third question about why we haven't changed our approach. It's because the medical way of thinking about and managing childbirth has become the norm. It has been widely accepted, and the ideas that relate to it have become deeply embedded in our culture. Despite there being little evidence for some of what we do, despite the value of not intervening unless there's a genuine medical reason, and despite the fact that interference often does more harm than good, we routinely monitor, manage and interfere in pregnancy and childbirth.

There is so much evidence to support the idea that we should change our approach. But some people have a vested interest in maintaining the status quo. It's possible, for instance, for health professionals and researchers to build their career around carrying out induction research. If your income is reliant on research funding, you might not want to challenge or speak out against the theories that you're researching. If your salary is partly paid by companies that manufacture and sell induction drugs or technologies, or if you have shares in those companies, then you might not be very inclined to want to limit their use.

But another part of the issue is that not everyone knows enough about the history of the ideas that have shaped our modern approach to birth. I'd like to change that.

Why ideas matter

As I write this book, we are living through a period in history that is described as late modern or postmodern. Yes, we use the term 'modern' to mean other things in everyday conversation too, but people who study history and culture use modern to describe the period from about the seventeenth century to now. That time has seen significant advances in science and technology, and changes in political ideas, as well as changes to how we move around the world and connect with each other.

Our culture (that is, the beliefs, ideas, customs and behaviours that we generally accept as 'the norm') is based on ideas that emerged from this period of great change and influence. The modern era encompasses and includes the scientific revolution, the Enlightenment and then the industrial revolution. These movements have led to us prioritising some ideas and ways of thinking over others. It's now well understood, however, that not all of the ideas, trends, norms and cultural changes that emerged from this period in history are good ones. The impact of human actions on the climate is just one illustration of this.

Many people across many fields now better understand some of what has happened, how it influences the world today and why we need to make significant changes. I am one of the people who has researched that in relation to childbirth, so let me try to explain exactly what some of these ideas are and how they are not always helpful and do not always promote women's, babies' and families' health.

How birth moved from home to hospital

For most of history, women have given birth at home. Their definition of home might vary a bit from ours, but the real point is that the idea of moving to a hospital to give birth is a relatively new one. Because of this, everyone alive today is the product of thousands of generations of families who have had successful home births. Even if your mother or grandmother had a more medicalised birth, their mothers and grandmothers almost certainly didn't.

Several decades ago, women in high-income countries began to go to hospital to give birth instead. The move to hospital birth was a response to beliefs about the value of nature, woman's bodies and birth, and the idea that these should be monitored and managed. The medical approach to childbirth in general has now become the norm (van Teijlingen 2005). Mostly, women go to hospital because they have been told that it is safer and, understandably, they want to do what's best for their baby. In the UK, the main move from home to hospital birth happened between the 1950s and the 1970s. It happened earlier in the USA and later in some European countries. Over time, services in many countries have become more and more centralised in big hospitals (Kirkham 2019), which raises another set of issues that I don't have space to discuss further here. But the ideas used to support this initial change were similar everywhere. In the UK, several government reports, influenced by medical men, said that hospital birth was safer than home birth (Ministry of Health 1970), and people understandably trusted that this was true.

But in the 1970s a Scottish statistician began to look more closely at the data that were underpinning the government documents and spotted a problem (Tew 1998). Professor Marjorie Tew was a statistician who taught statistics to medical students. While looking at some of the birth surveys produced in the 1970s, she realised that what the medical profession was saying about the safety of home and hospital birth was not actually supported by the data. When she analysed these data, she realised that hospital wasn't actually a safer place to give birth than home. She also realised that women were, perhaps accidentally, being given inaccurate information. As someone who was committed to both scientific rigour and good care for women, Tew was keen to bring this to light. Everyone is entitled to make mistakes, after all, and perhaps, she thought, the Government hadn't realised its mistake. So Tew wrote up her findings to share with colleagues in a medical journal and sent it off to the editor.

For years, British medical journals refused to publish her work. It took until 1985 for a journal (the Journal of the Royal College of General Practitioners) to publish the results of her analysis (Tew 1985). By this time, hospital birth was well established as the norm, and it was far too late to turn the tide. That hasn't stopped people trying, though. Marjorie Tew is one of a number of scientists, doctors, midwives, social scientists, activists and others who have fought and are continuing to fight for honesty and an evidence-based approach to childbirth. There was, and remains, a strong movement of people committed to women and families being able to access other perspectives on birth, and about the evidence that can help us understand what is and isn't beneficial. But despite their efforts and despite the evidence, most people still believe the message put out by the UK Government of the 1970s and by medical organisations around the world today. They believe that it's safer to give birth in hospital and to allow the birth process to be medically managed. But if you're healthy and don't have any medical conditions, that's not necessarily the case (Birthplace in England Collaborative Group 2011).

The technocratic paradigm

To save us spelling out long definitions every time, social scientists and other experts describe the modern approach to childbirth (and many other facets of life) as the technocratic paradigm. The word paradigm simply means a particular set of ideas, beliefs and practices. Sometimes we describe these ideas as the medical model or the obstetric approach. It's a particular way of thinking about the world and then acting on those beliefs.

People who take a technocratic approach to pregnancy and birth view childbirth as a potentially pathological and risk-laden process. They are likely to be scared of it. They believe that women and babies should be carefully monitored and managed via a series of interventions embedded within modern maternity care and that women should be told what to do and how to behave. A key feature of this approach is an almost complete lack of trust in women's bodies and in women's knowledge. Professionals and machines are deemed to 'know better,' as I'll discuss more in chapter four. In my own research, I describe the obstetric approach as one of 'process management' (Wickham 2008). That's because some people see pregnancy and birth literally as a process to be managed, a bit like in a factory. The woman is almost an incidental vessel or vehicle rather than the person at the centre of a potentially transformative, social, psychological, spiritual and physiological journey. Process management has led to standardisation, as Professor Mavis Kirkham shows:

"If a large organisation is to be run for maximum efficiency management control is required to monitor and ensure that efficiency. Midwives cannot be trusted to do midwifery or to decide a woman's care in response to her needs as this might lead to care being given beyond the 'efficient' norm. Thus standardisation is required. Standardisation requires care to be defined as a series of tasks which can be monitored rather than a continuing supportive relationship… Standardisation is justified as preventing really bad care but it also prevents really good care from being the norm; though many midwives strive to give good care, often at great cost to themselves. This approach is often described as being evidence-based, but research deals with the general, never stating what an individual needs and much evidence is based on a consensus of those thoroughly versed in cost-saving." (Kirkham 2019).

The technocratic paradigm is not the only way of thinking about pregnancy and birth. As you might already have gathered, I am more inclined to focus on the woman's journey. Like many holistic midwives, when I'm on call for a birth, my car boot is full of equipment and I am highly skilled in using emergency procedures on the occasions when things do unexpectedly go wrong. But I keep those skills tucked away and do everything I can to optimise the conditions for physiological birth. Many other people believe in this more holistic approach too. But we're not in the majority. Despite the lack of evidence to support it (as I will be discussing in later chapters as well as this one), the technocratic approach is the dominant one in many high- and middle-income countries and it is increasingly being adopted in low-income countries as well.

It's important to understand that not all obstetricians, employed midwives or other health professionals take a technocratic approach or fully subscribe to this belief system. Some do, some don't, and most of us are far too interesting and human and complex to have our ideas put in one box with a particular label on it, thank you very much! Those of us who try to research, describe and write about the world need to create categories and name things in order to be able to discuss them. But the world is actually messier than that.

It's not accurate or helpful to make generalisations and assumptions that directly link beliefs or attitudes to professional or occupational groups. Yes, the obstetric belief system is shared by many obstetricians. But some are working hard to change it, and don't subscribe to it at all (Barrett 2014, Small 2020). Many employed midwives are in the difficult position of not wanting to go along with it but find that resistance isn't compatible with keeping their job or earning a living so they can feed their children. The system is far bigger than they are. That's partly because the ideas that form the technocratic paradigm are deeply embedded in our culture. The ideas are embraced by many people who have never set foot in a maternity hospital, and they permeate almost every aspect of our lives. I also sometimes hear people working at the more alternative end of the spectrum promoting some of the key ideas of the technocratic paradigm and in some cases undermining women's rights. Many women and families strongly believe in these ideas too. It's important to bear in mind, when we talk about the belief systems like the medical model, the technocratic approach, or the obstetric paradigm, that we're talking about a set of beliefs and practices, and that these beliefs and practices aren't directly and only linked to one particular professional or occupational group.

Women aren't machines

I've already explained that the belief system that we refer to as the technocratic paradigm is rooted in some of the ideas which emerged from the Enlightenment era. At that time, philosophers and scientists were creating a model of their ideas about how the universe worked. They decided that:

"…the universe is mechanistic, following predictable laws which those enlightened enough to free themselves from the limitations of medieval superstition could discover through science and manipulate through technology in order to decrease their dependence on nature." (Davis-Floyd 1993: 299).

In simple terms, the idea is that everything in the universe is like a machine. Never mind nature's rhythms, seasons and cycles, which are abundant and unmissable even if you live in the most modern of cities. There is a rhythm to the year which we can see in the sun and moon and in the plants and trees around us. Women's bodies have a clear monthly cycle, and there is also a rhythm to pregnancy and other seasons of women's lives. But for those who believe in the technocratic paradigm, this is irrelevant. Everything is like a machine, and this includes all aspects of nature, including our bodies. So, in theory, if you study bodies (or earthquakes or squirrels) well enough, you can create a sort of user manual of rules and guidelines (like the one that comes with a car) and always predict what they will do.

Nice idea, especially if you're the kind of person who likes to feel in control. No evidence that it's true, though. In fact, there's evidence all around us that it isn't. Along with many other things in the universe, like the weather, the timing of when we're hungry, tired or need to go to the loo, and why there's never any sign of what the problem was when you finally reach the end of a motorway traffic jam, our bodies are often mysterious and not very predictable. Yes, we can sometimes make a guess. But we're often wrong, and sometimes the best we can do is to talk about probabilities. We might be able to say, for instance, that you have a ninety per cent chance of this, or a ten per cent chance of that. Or that one in a thousand babies will have difficulties. But we have no way of knowing or predicting which one.

Physicists and mathematicians realised that the universe wasn't mechanistic a long time ago, and they've adapted their thinking. They embrace uncertainty in many different ways and understand that things are far more complex and interesting than we once thought. But this understanding is taking longer to trickle down into other areas of life, including many areas of medicine, health and birth. So obstetrics claims to be scientific but some of its core ideas are rooted in a three-hundred-year-old theory that scientists now know isn't true.

It gets worse, though. The not-very-accurate idea of the universe being mechanistic is also linked with some other beliefs that we're still hanging on to, despite them not being true or helpful either. One is the idea of reductionism. This is an approach where people thought that the best way to study and understand complex systems (like the human body, or the process of birth) was to separate them out and/or reduce them to simpler components. Or to focus on one aspect, like someone's age, size or race, and to ignore everything else about their health. I'll look at that more in chapter seven.

As you might know, the French philosopher René Descartes pronounced that it was possible to separate the mind and body. As you might also know, this doesn't reflect reality. In birth, we see the evidence of this when we look at how the wider environment of birth can affect the woman's hormones and thus the progress of her labour (Daviss & Johnson 1998, Gaskin 2004, Wickham 2009a). I have heard hundreds of stories of women whose labours were affected by social, psychological and environmental aspects. Like Jemima, who went into labour just minutes after her stressed husband got on a plane to fly to a conference in another city, leaving her finally feeling relaxed enough to let go. She gave birth before he had landed, and it turned out that they were both immensely relieved that things had happened that way.

I've also seen many women hold onto their babies until they feel safe, in the broadest sense of the word. Sometimes, that means getting away from people who want to interfere. One of my favourite stories is about Camille, who was in two minds about what to do, but eventually decided to go to an antenatal ward for monitoring of her 42-week pregnancy. Her main reason for going was to avoid negative repercussions from being labelled as a 'bad mother,' which is terrible, but that's another conversation.

Camille had been having a few contractions on the journey to the hospital, but, unsurprisingly to her midwife, that all stopped the moment she stepped through the hospital door. They restarted on the journey home and her family didn't even manage to fill the birth pool before she gave birth. To save you wondering, I should tell you that their efforts weren't wasted, as she had a nice long bath in it that evening with her newborn baby.

The moral of this and the thousands of similar stories that women, midwives and birth workers can tell you is that our minds affect our bodies all the time, and vice versa. Sometimes labour can start, as it did with Carrie, and then stop if someone feels unsafe. In other situations, emotional or social issues can delay the start of labour.

"I've seen labour postponed by stress, rough jagged relationships, fear or a family tragedy, definitely by lack of sex!" (Amy, midwife).

If a woman's labour stops when she enters a hospital, the logical conclusion from a woman-centred perspective is to consider that perhaps the woman doesn't feel safe in the hospital and a change of environment is warranted. Maybe she needs a different caregiver as well. But what actually happens in our modern culture is that she is told that her body is failing to labour adequately. She's then subjected to intervention to make her body 'behave' according to the mechanistic mathematical principles that the people who take a technocratic approach would like nature to obey. This intervention may or may not work. It may lead to more intervention. It sometimes leads to the woman or baby suffering distress and needing to be 'rescued' from their plight, perhaps by a caesarean section. Then, to add insult to injury, many of those in whom intervention is overused are sent home thinking that their or their babies' lives were saved by it, when that's not the tiniest bit true.

It's not true that we can separate out our mind, body and spirit (whatever that means to you) from each other and from the wider environment. Yet it's one of the fundamental beliefs on which the technocratic viewpoint is based.

Just to be clear, though, I'm not suggesting for a moment that complications never occur naturally. They totally do. I'm also not arguing that intervention is always the cause of complications, or that it's never beneficial. That's rubbish. Sometimes, it's genuinely life-saving. But it's often overused, and that causes harm to women, babies and families.

Separation does more harm than good

The obstetric worldview contains other problematic ideas as well. Its proponents tend to see things in a linear fashion. It doesn't generally acknowledge complexity, and has a strong attachment to the idea of mathematical certainty. Again, science itself has moved on from some of these ideas, but some branches of medicine haven't, and obstetrics is one of them.

Separation, for example, remains an ongoing theme. Practitioners are still encouraged to distance themselves emotionally from the women they attend. Women who give birth in hospital are separated from their lives and families. If they agree to induction, they can sometimes be on an antenatal or induction ward for several days while labour gets going, but without their partners or birth supporters. This was especially true throughout the pandemic.

Several social scientists have looked at this issue of separation and how, over the past half century or more, newborn babies have been separated from their mothers by means of a number of obstetric practices and technologies (Katz Rothman 1982, 1984, Davis-Floyd 1992). They often see how, even when our instincts tell us otherwise, we are persuaded to hand our babies over, following social norms. So much of what we see and hear (including what's on the TV, as George's words at the beginning of the chapter illustrated) somehow gets us to accept that having our babies weighed and measured and injected with medicines is more important than them having their first cuddle with us. Skin-to-skin (or, as my hairy-chested friend Matt once called it, skin-to-fur) contact with our mother straight after birth brings many benefits and helps babies adapt to life outside the womb (Unicef 2021).

Can you really imagine another mammal, say a wolf or an orangutan, allowing someone to take their newborn away? Thinking about how an animal would respond can highlight two things. The first is what the mammalian instinct likely tells us to do. The second is how such strong instincts can be so overridden by cultural ideas. That in itself is good enough reason to think hard about the ideas that are embedded in our culture and whether they are truly serving us.

In fact, when they think about these things, many people realise that they don't serve us or our humanity and that they can do more harm than good. They're right. Enlightenment ideas aren't very people-centred. Neither are they nature friendly or sustainable. We're not machines, separation isn't a good thing, and we shouldn't be managed as if we were items on a factory assembly line. More than this, some of these ideas, and the way that they interfere with 'what nature intended' can be harmful. Yet, within the technocratic paradigm, birth is seen as a production process and the female body has come to be seen as a defective machine which needs to be monitored and controlled.

Babies aren't end products

In a system which deals with thousands of births every year and is based on ideas that emerged from the industrial era, babies tend to be seen as the 'end product.' In fact, the 'end product' of a live baby, with a focus on the immediate physical outcomes, has become the key marker of success and the priority of obstetric management of the birth process.

Now, I'm not saying for a moment that having a live baby isn't important. It clearly is. But it's not the only thing that matters. It's also important to have a healthy mother, who feels confident and isn't traumatised by the unnecessary measures taken to try and ensure that the baby is well. And it's no good if the measures that we take to attempt to keep more babies alive at birth lead to poorer health later on which causes some of them to become sick and die before their first birthday, as I discussed in chapter one.

We need to look not just at the immediate, short-term physical health of the baby, but at the medium- and long-term health of the mother and baby in the widest possible sense. If an intervention might save one extra baby in a thousand but puts them at higher risk of ill health and other problems later, is that justified? If something will save one baby but leave three hundred women injured, disappointed or traumatised and two hundred of the babies with medium- and long-term health issues, is that justifiable? Some people who think in technocratic, production line terms are certain that it is. That's because they're focused only on what happens at the end of the process of birth, and they don't think or look beyond that.

Some of our knowledge in this area came from sociologist Ann Oakley. She found that one of the features of the obstetric frame of reference was, *"...the selection of limited criteria of reproductive success, i.e. perinatal and maternal mortality rates."* (Oakley 1980: 10). In other words, she showed that medicine was focusing only on short-term, immediate outcomes, like stillbirth and Apgar scores, which are a measure of the baby's physical wellbeing straight after birth, and not on the long-term consequences of particular decisions. The technocratic approach doesn't look at the bigger picture and thus doesn't allow people to take everything into account so that they can make the decisions that are right for them and their family. After all, it is they who will be living with the consequences.

It's also important to remember that our predictions are based only on probability, and there's no certainty here. We can't tell you ahead of time if you're the one in a thousand, or one of the nine hundred and ninety-nine. The Enlightenment idea of certainty is very appealing, but sadly it's a fantasy.

The ideas that I'm sharing in this chapter have been discussed by a number of social scientists. If you'd like to read about this area in more depth, look at the work of Ann Oakley (1980, 1984, 1993), Barbara Katz Rothman (1982, 1984), Robbie Davis-Floyd (1992) and Jo Murphy-Lawless (1998).

In simple terms, the ideas that emerged from the Enlightenment have led people to believe that birth is a process that can and should be contained and controlled. But the journey of birth is not predictable, and trying to control pregnancy and birth can lead to harm because of the suppression of natural rhythms and processes which have evolved to be beneficial for women and babies.

Attempts to control birth can also be oppressive and coercive to women, which I'll come to later in this chapter. The technocratic approach has convinced us that we can and should control pregnant and birthing bodies. We should monitor them, manage them and, if we think things aren't going as they should, then we should intervene and try to manipulate what's happening.

But there's another important idea that emerged from the Enlightenment and it has become the key to how all of this monitoring, management and manipulation is justified. That idea is something we call 'risk.'

Birth as risky business

There's a very specific reason why the obstetric paradigm has been able to justify controlling women's bodies. In a nutshell, the people who promote the obstetric approach to birth make two linked claims. The first of these claims, as I've said, is that pregnancy and birth are risky, and therefore need to be closely managed. The second claim is that proponents of the obstetric paradigm are the people best placed to manage the risk and to create the rules (such as the due date and the recommendation for induction) which dictate how women's and babies' bodies should be monitored and managed.

Sociologists have been unpacking the idea of managing risk for several decades now, as Ann Oakley shows:

"Two kinds of strategies have been especially important in establishing the rationale of modern antenatal care. One relates to the medical-professional claim to know what is going on in the uterus better than the mother herself, and the other refers to the notion of controlling the termination of pregnancy – the onset of labour." (Oakley 1984: 27)

As another sociologist, Jo Murphy-Lawless (1998) writes, women have always understood that childbirth is potentially dangerous, and they have always accepted this. Life is risky. But she also shows how the idea of risk has been co-opted to justify medical control of childbirth.

"The question of risk has been a constant reference point for obstetrics whenever there has been a controversy over who should control the birth process, women or medicine." (Murphy-Lawless 1998: 21)

Many professionals are fed up with the focus on risk.

"Risk, it really steals the joy out of situations." (Kim, midwife).

"There's no joy anymore. There should be ... there's the potential for so much joy. Birth should be one of the most joyful experiences we have. It can be. But it seems like you can only be sure of that if you go outside the system to do it, and avoid the risk narrative that's embedded within it these days." (Kerry, midwife).

But professionals working in modern health care systems have very little choice but to focus on risk. Because it is such a key aspect of the medical approach, the idea of risk is built into everything that professionals do as part of their work. It's not necessarily that people are deliberately using the notion of risk with the intention of controlling women and families. In some cases, health professionals genuinely fear that something terrible might happen, even if the evidence shows otherwise. Having a medical or midwifery degree doesn't immunise you against having a poor understanding of risk, or against being overly and inappropriately influenced by your experiences, your education or by the ideas of our time.

We live in a litigious society, and many maternity care professionals face legal action at least once in their career. People understandably fear reprisal and the loss of their career. It's scary, especially when you've done your best, and I speak from experience. The way our modern legal system works means that professionals will always get into more trouble for the things they didn't do rather than the things they did. That's another reason why there's too much intervention, despite the evidence that it's generally better to leave well alone unless there is good reason to interfere.

It's also important to remember that some health professionals don't get to see gentle, physiological births. Most obstetricians don't see the women who quietly turn up at midnight, give birth in the capable care of the labour ward or co-located midwife-led birth centre midwives with the door closed and then go home a few hours later. Doctors don't tend to get called to straightforward births. The births they attend are those where the woman and/or her baby are perceived to be running into difficulties.

If all you see are the situations where things go wrong, and you're a normal human who has a brain that is hard-wired to look for risk and try to keep yourself safe, that's where you'll put your focus. That's what you'll worry about. That's what you'll try to prevent; maybe even if there's no evidence that prevention efforts are effective. *At least you're doing something.*

Risk management lacks logic

The thing is, of course, that women's bodies are individual, variable and complex. They don't always respond well to attempts to control them. Especially when the attempts at control happen in an environment that isn't conducive to the hormones that orchestrate birth. Our bodies are also linked to minds that may sense that the environment isn't safe for us (though this isn't necessarily something that people are aware of) and they can respond by stopping the process of labour. That's exactly what happened in the story I told about how Camille's labour stopped as soon as she entered the hospital. Her body was protecting her from what she felt (perhaps subconsciously) was an unsafe environment.

A similar problem occurs when we consider the situation where a woman's labour hasn't started by the time that the obstetric paradigm thinks it ought to. Women and families are told that their baby is 'at risk'; that their baby may not make it if they don't agree to induction. As I discuss throughout this book, these claims are often not based on good evidence and they often lack logic. But, in a situation where people believe in all the ideas that I've discussed in this chapter and feel compelled (perhaps because of social norms and pressure from others) to agree, that doesn't matter. If people accept the authority of the medical model, they'll tend to follow the recommendations that are made. Who wants to take the chance of disagreeing with an obstetric recommendation and then being the one in a thousand who doesn't have a live, healthy baby at the end of the day? The threat of risk is immeasurably powerful. Once the idea of risk is introduced, it can be overwhelming and sometimes irresistible, even for those women and families who don't believe in the technocratic approach (Machin & Scammell 1997). And yet these threats are often biased, inappropriate, sometimes baseless, and not inclusive of the bigger picture.

"He [the consultant obstetrician] *said, just imagine what might have happened if you had been at home ... if things had gone wrong. And I thought, well if I had stayed at home then none of this*

would have happened. You wouldn't have been able to do the episiotomy [that] *left me incontinent, that I still have nightmares about because you didn't listen when I said no. I might not have had postnatal depression. I might have enjoyed ... the first eight months of* [my baby's] *life. None of that would have happened if I had stayed home. But I went along with him because he said my baby would die if I didn't."* (Chloe).

This is seen in what women are told about induction, too.

"I was frightened into induction with the scary statistics. Had many complications. Wish I had said no." (Padya).

"I was so annoyed that once I went past 40 weeks how quickly the doctors/consultants wanted to highlight all the risks associated with going "overdue" but not one of them would be honest when I asked about the risks involved with induction. They didn't want to talk about that." (Mabel).

"After a wonderful pregnancy I was told about induction at 38 weeks simply because I had my 40th birthday a month before my due date. I pointed out to various midwives that perhaps the fact that I'm a healthy non-smoker, was active throughout pregnancy, had immaculate blood tests would have made a difference but they said those were the numbers. That someone had to be those numbers and it's up to you but do you want to accept the risk? I accepted, not happy, and had the worst birth experience I could imagine. I left the hospital with a healthy baby but we were so traumatised that it took a long time to recover and even to establish breast feeding. I felt robbed of a once in a lifetime experience." (Anna).

The risks of the obstetric approach

But there's an even bigger problem. Many of the people who have analysed the obstetric approach to childbirth point out that, ironically, the obstetric approach itself poses risks to women and babies. The medical paradigm sees risk as 'the enemy' and itself as the means to ensure safety in childbirth. Research, however, has consistently demonstrated that obstetric intervention causes harm, especially when it is overused (Oakley 1984, 1993, Tew 1985, 1986, Enkin *et al* 2000,

Wagner 2006, Gibbons *et al* 2010, Miller 2016, Nelson *et al* 2016, Çalik *et al* 2018, Seijmonsbergen-Schermers *et al* 2019, 2020, Dahlen *et al* 2021). Many other studies have shown the downsides of the (over)medicalised approach during the past few decades.

There is a long history of challenges to the obstetric approach to the management of birth in general and induction in particular. As well as those already mentioned, Ann Cartwright (1979), Sally Inch (1982), Sheila Kitzinger (1987) and Beverley Beech (1987) all raised questions about induction of labour in the UK in the years when this was becoming entrenched as an intervention. They and many others around the world have sought, and still seek, to inform women of the pros and cons of induction of labour as well as the fact that they have a right to decline.

The obstetric approach is also often seen as oppressive to women, and to women's knowledge. As Edwards and Murphy-Lawless (2006) discuss, *"...science and medicine have already mapped out what women's 'responsible' decisions should be in order to reduce risk"* (37). In other words, women are often forced, either directly or indirectly, into particular childbirth choices because of the power of the medical model.

In our culture, medical knowledge is deemed to be far more valuable than women's own knowledge. As one sociologist noted: *"...women are not heard within obstetric space. We have no authorised knowledge claims."* (Murphy-Lawless 1998: 254-55). So a woman might intuitively feel that her baby needs longer in the womb, that the due date is incorrect or that the ultrasound is wrong about her baby being 'too big.' But this kind of knowledge doesn't count. It's not generally considered valid within technocratic systems of maternity care. In some areas, women are listened to and well supported no matter what their decision. In others, if a woman wants to make decisions that are outside the guidelines, she may have to either battle, or seek alternative options.

Birth and time

In current obstetrics, the notion of women going into labour and giving birth in their own time is becoming unusual. The ideas embedded in the obstetric paradigm have come to form a set of generally accepted boundaries. These boundaries dictate what those who embrace the medical model of birth see as the appropriate length of pregnancy and labour. These boundaries are now embedded in many guidelines (e.g. ACOG 2021, NICE 2021b) but, as I'll discuss further in later chapters, just as with the move to hospital birth a few decades ago, the guidelines aren't always supported by good evidence.

Like the concept of risk, our modern ideas about time have roots in older ideas. You may have heard of Pythagoras, who suggested that number and measure were timeless truths (Seife 2000). You might also know that Sir Isaac Newton's work heavily influenced the scientific revolution. He used time as an absolute and independent variable within his mechanics and that still influences the way we think today. But many of our current ideas about time came out of the later industrial revolution. Time has been linked with efficiency and productivity. We live in a culture which sees being overdue as a bad thing (which also helps reinforce obstetric ideas about the end of pregnancy) and modern western culture is focused on speed, tasks, schedules and procedures (Hall 1984). The clock is deemed a *"…crucial organising principle in industrial society."* (Helman 1987: 969).

Time is also a key feature in health care systems, and I don't just mean the clock that is on every hospital labour room wall, which causes some women to feel incredibly pressured. (Top tip: cover it with a towel or tee-shirt or, if someone can reach it, take the battery out. Or just turn the lights out so you can't see it.) Time is used to measure how well staff members, wards, hospitals and systems are functioning, for instance in relation to waiting times for diagnosis and treatment. It's used to arrange our working lives. We 'clock in' and 'clock out,' and time dictates the duties of workers via shift patterns. We're so used to it organising us that we barely notice how much it impacts our lives, creating a sense that we have to hurry everywhere, that certain things must happen by a certain time, even though usually nothing bad will happen if they don't. Is it so unthinkable that some patients could bathe in the evenings rather than by 10am? After all, some people prefer to shower before getting into bed at home. When we take a step back and ask some of these questions, we can see that time is indeed used as a crucial organising principle and yet there is often no good reason for this.

Within the obstetric approach to childbirth, time is also seen as a crucial means of measuring women's progress through pregnancy and birth. Many of the holistic midwives who I've worked with and carried out research with over the years take a different approach. They don't ignore time altogether, but they focus just as much on wellbeing. They are much more accepting of and interested in natural rhythms. The rhythms of a woman's body and of her environment. The rhythm and pattern that her immediate maternal ancestors' births followed. How her own previous birth experiences played out.

But most women don't get to think about their experiences and births in this way. The dominance of the technocratic approach means that many people don't think twice about immediately asking women when their baby is due, as if this is the most important thing to know. Most women have been taught to believe that medical timeframes are a more valid way of deciding when their baby should be born than their own body or baby. Concepts like pre-term, term and post-term and the medical focus on the estimated due date are all examples of how obstetric temporal (or time) norms have become superimposed upon women's bodies and on our experiences. They arose out of the ideas that I've discussed in this chapter; the industrial approach of the production line, process management and the baby as an end product. They have become deeply embedded in our culture. They can be heard in the language and concepts that we hear and see every day. They separate what obstetrics sees as 'normal' and 'not normal', even though (as I'll discuss more in later chapters) those categories aren't based on good evidence either. They reflect the focus on risk.

But they don't reflect women's and midwives' knowledge and experiences, or the wider evidence that we have about birth. Left to themselves, women's bodies would dance and birth to their own rhythm, although this might not be one easily mapped onto two-dimensional, linear charts like the partograms used in maternity systems to chart the physical progress of some aspects a woman's labour. These medical concepts don't reflect the reality of how Camille's and Jemima's bodies instinctively waited until the time was right. Neither do they reflect the wonder in George's eyes; the awe which arose from the sight of seeing a woman birth in her own power and in her own time.

3. Guidelines, evidence and listening to women

In May 2021, the National Institute for Health and Care Excellence (NICE) published the draft of a proposed new guideline on inducing labour (NICE 2021a). NICE is the body that provides national guidance and advice to inform health and social care in the UK. Many other countries look to the NICE guidance to inform practice and policy as well.

The new draft guideline related to, *"…the circumstances, methods and monitoring for inducing labour in pregnant women."* (NICE 2021a: 1). It caused significant concern among women, families, midwives, doctors, birth workers and others, and numerous individuals and organisations sprang into action to respond to NICE and share their many questions and issues with the proposed guidance. That's because it contained some recommendations that weren't evidence-based, but which would have impacted significantly on women's experiences and decision making, and could cause serious problems for maternity care and service providers.

Thankfully, the final version of the guidance (NICE 2021b) did not contain all of the recommendations that were initially proposed in the draft. But concerns remain. The new guidance is not explicitly clear in some areas, which will lead to it being interpreted differently in different areas and hospitals. It contains statements and recommendations which undermine the idea that women's and babies' bodies are, on the whole, capable of determining when labour should begin. There are contradictions between this guidance and some of the other documents that inform maternity practice. As a result, healthy, low-risk women will still be offered induction, as Julie Frohlich describes so well in the foreword to this book. In this chapter, I'm going to look in more depth at some of the reasons why people are worried about induction guidelines, and discuss the growing body of evidence we have about how induction guidelines and practices affect women and families.

The 'offer' of induction

Until recently, spontaneous labour was considered to be the norm and induction was only offered in some very specific circumstances. In the years preceding the 2021 NICE guidance, induction had been offered more liberally, and concern about this had been growing. But the biggest overall issue with the 2021 NICE guideline which caused so much controversy was that it further cemented a significant shift towards discussing induction with all women. New proposed recommendations include mentioning induction earlier in pregnancy and offering membrane sweeping at 39 weeks. The draft guidance also recommended offering earlier induction, at 39 weeks of pregnancy, for certain groups of women simply because they were perceived to be 'at higher risk.' As I will discuss below, that particular recommendation was removed from the final guidance, but the shift towards normalising induction of labour as a reasonable and normal way to end pregnancy for many women still remains.

Sometimes, when I say or write this, people point out that the guideline isn't the law. This is true. As long as they have mental capacity, no-one has to agree to the treatment or care that a guideline, midwife or doctor offers or recommends. People point out that the guideline uses terms like, *'offered,'* and *'should be considered,'* which are not absolute statements. This shows that everybody has a choice, they say, and so therefore surely it is a good thing that induction is there as an offer for those who need or want it, and those who don't want it can just decline? They make it sound like when a waiter brings the pepper mill to the table when your pasta is served. Pepper or no pepper? Your choice.

But, although some people talk about maternity choices as if they are similar to other choices we make as consumers, like whether we like white or brown bread, or if we'll buy the red or blue shoes or think about it and come back later, they are not like this in reality, for a number of reasons.

Many people do not know or understand that induction is

the woman's decision or just an 'offer.' Induction is often presented as a given, or an assumption. As these two women's words show, this may be quite subtle.

"My issue is they don't talk to you and make a plan with you like they're supposed to, they tell you what you're doing and for some women what a doctor or midwife says is gospel and it's not always the case. Women don't realise that everything is your choice from the way you give birth to even having scans. It needs to be common knowledge for all women that what you want and how you want it is paramount." (Nike).

"I was booked for induction, due to going over my due date. I was terrified about it ending up with me having a c-section etc, so I just phoned them up and said I'm not coming in. They were fine with it. I went into natural labour the next day, but there very much was an assumption that I would have an induction." (Sophia).

Another issue is the way that induction and some other interventions are discussed by some care providers. Let me first note though that there are some people offering good, respectful care. They strive to give evidence-based information (which is a challenging task when the guidelines on which they are expected to base their practice are not actually always evidence-based), and they make it clear that induction is just one option. But not everybody takes this approach. Some care providers actively coerce women into having labour induced, sometimes by using scare tactics. Others stand by while their colleagues do this. Some don't (or feel they can't) offer information, even when they can see that women and families haven't been properly informed about the evidence or the individual situation they are in. This woman's words are sadly just one example of something I hear almost every day:

"I felt forced into induction. I'd had sweeps and was 2-3cm dilated, and was as sure as I could be that it would happen in good time. I had a scan at 42 weeks and the doctor was awful. Nothing was wrong but she insisted I should be induced as [she claimed] *'the risk of stillbirth increases exponentially.' I reluctantly agreed to go in for induction the next day."* (Sal).

In case you are not aware, I want to clarify that the risk of stillbirth does not increase exponentially. This is an untrue statement made by someone who clearly doesn't understand maths, let alone the evidence base around induction of labour. Sadly, I hear from many women and families who have been told that they have *"a high chance of stillbirth,"* or that their baby, *"…will almost certainly die if you don't come in for induction right away,"* when this is absolutely not true. Sheila Kitzinger (2006) described this as *"emotional blackmail,"* and many people refer to it as *"playing the dead baby card"* (Wickham 2018a, 2019). It's really important that we name and discuss this, as so many women and families encounter it.

One thing to remember is that, if a care provider really was that worried about your baby, they wouldn't be offering induction, which often takes three days to get going. If they were that worried, or if the risk was really high, they would and should be offering an immediate caesarean section.

Just one of the knock-on effects of the use of scare tactics is that those who believe what they have been told and agree to an induction are then terrified when they are then told that they need to be rescheduled for later in the week because there are no beds. Or when (as is often the case) theirs is one of the induced labours that takes three days to start. As one woman who was in that situation told me years later, *"I felt like a ticking time bomb, and it was horrible. Only years later did I find out it wasn't true. Now I can never get that time back. It will stay with me forever."* (Lou).

I will discuss the actual difference in risk and the statistics relating to this area (which are far different from this, and there is no exponential increase anywhere) in later chapters. That's because it's important to look at the statistics in relation to the reason that's given for induction, though it's also vital to take the bigger picture of the woman's and baby's health and wellbeing into account as well. The point I want to make here is that some health care providers do use coercion. Sometimes in a very friendly, caring tone and with a smile on their face. Some believe what they're saying, and some are aware that they are misleading you. But when health care providers are doing this, it is next to impossible for women and families to make a decision based upon the evidence and their individual circumstances.

In the current climate, maternity care options are nothing like restaurant menu options. Because it's as if the waiter brings the pepper and says, *"…well, it's up to you, of course, and I understand you don't like pepper, but the meal could be poisonous, and there's a high chance that your unborn baby will die if you don't let me grind the pepper on it."* It's clearly a ridiculous statement, but will you be having pepper now?

Why 'the norm' matters

There are other reasons why we need to be careful about what guidelines are offering as the default option or standard of care. Women and families might not speak good English (or whatever language their care is being offered in) or understand that they even have options. Women may be fearful of medical staff, even in situations where the medical staff are totally woman-centred. Disobedience or questioning authority is often discouraged and some women come from cultures or countries where this is punished. They may fear that they will not be cared for as well if they are 'stroppy' or make decisions that go against the grain. That is, sadly, something I hear often from Black and Brown women. Some people have a partner who doesn't want to step outside the norm. One of the biggest issues is that, as I noted in chapter one, many people assume that, *'what is, must be best.'* For all these reasons and many more, most people will go along with the norm. This is why it's crucially important that we ensure that the norm – or what's in the guideline – spells out the best standard of care, based on the best available evidence which takes as many factors as possible into account, including women's knowledge, views and experiences.

The problems with the draft guideline

I mentioned above that the 2021 guideline contains the recommendation that induction should be discussed early in pregnancy and that membrane sweeping be offered after 39+0 weeks. Many women are offered or given an induction date and told about membrane sweeping even sooner than this. It's important to consider what effect introducing the topic of induction might do to women's confidence, especially when this happens early in pregnancy and is then repeated. Because offering membrane sweeping from 39 weeks undermines the idea that women's bodies are entirely capable of going into labour on their own without routine intervention. It's a little like standing at the bottom of a hill to let fit, healthy people who are about to climb it know that a helicopter is hovering, ready to pick them up and take them to the top if they can't manage it. The very confident people might laugh that off. Some of the less confident might feel relieved. And some – and this is a key concern – who were previously unworried may start to doubt their own ability. Why would a helicopter be hovering if people were confident in your ability to get to the top? Do they know something you don't? As we know from chapters one and two, the mind and body are connected and the hormones of birth can be influenced by a woman's mind and wider environment. This can have a significant effect on some women. Early discussions of induction and offers of induction interventions can also leave people feeling that their care providers don't have confidence in their ability to labour and birth without help.

As I wrote above, one recommendation which was in the draft guidance was of particular concern to many of those who responded to NICE. I want to look at this more closely, even though it was removed from the final version of the guideline. That's because it relates to groups of women who are already being offered induction simply because they are deemed to be at higher risk. The offer of induction is made despite there being little to no evidence that induction of labour will benefit them or their babies, as I will discuss in later chapters. The draft (NICE 2021a) guideline had recommended that practitioners:

"Consider induction of labour from 39+0 weeks in women with otherwise uncomplicated singleton pregnancies who are at a higher risk of complications associated with continued pregnancy (for example, BMI 30 kg/m2 23 or above, age 35 years or above, with a black, Asian or minority ethnic family background, or after assisted conception)." (NICE 2021a: 6). None of this is evidence based.

Many of those who responded to the draft NICE guidance – including myself – were concerned about two related things. The first was the evidence on which the recommendations were based. In some cases, statements about 'the evidence' were not supported by a reference. When one clicked the links in the document in an attempt to see the evidence, the recommendation turned out to be based on the *"knowledge and experience"* of the panel. It seems inadequate to base national guidance that impacts so many women and babies and that has potential to harm as well as benefit on the panel's knowledge and expertise, valuable as that may be. This is very different from basing guidance on clear, robust evidence drawn from carefully designed research. In some instances, there was evidence but it hadn't been included.

As the lead authors of the Royal College of Midwives' (RCM) response to the draft guidance wrote:

"The care midwives provide needs to be informed by the very best evidence available and should not be limited to randomised controlled trials as seems the case with this guideline. There are some good observational studies, as well as qualitative reviews that can offer data on the long-term outcomes for women and babies, including the impact on mental health and their experience of care." (Brigante & Harlev-Lam 2021).

The second concern about the draft guidance was that it seemed to completely ignore the experiences of women and the fact that a growing body of research is showing that many women have concerns about induction. It's important to bear in mind that the draft NICE (2021a) guidance also came on top of concerns about shifts in practice that had occurred during the coronavirus pandemic.

"Since the start of the COVID-19 pandemic ... stories have emerged ... of women having their labor induced, being forced to have cesarean sections, giving birth alone, and being separated from their babies immediately after birth. Current responses to the pandemic in maternal healthcare and the acceptance of these measures on the basis of "necessity" not only imply serious infringements of human rights but also present a serious risk that the precarious status of women's rights in childbirth will become the new normal." (Drandić & van Leeuwen 2020).

Researchers had recently undertaken a national survey, *"...to examine whether and how the COVID-19 pandemic has changed practice around IOL in the UK."* (Harkness *et al* 2021). Senior midwives and obstetricians completed an online survey, which showed that some Trusts and Health Boards had changed aspects of their induction practice without consultation or evidence for this. Some had changed the method of induction, some the criteria for who could return home during the early stages of induction. The authors noted that, *"Much of the change was reported as happening in response to attempts to minimise hospital attendance and restrictions on birth partners accompanying women."* (Harkness *et al* 2021).

The same study showed that the average induction rate in the Trusts and Boards that responded was 34%; just over a third of all women. Some Trusts and Boards had induction rates of more than 40%, and a couple had rates far higher.

Respondents in Harkness *et al*'s (2021) research were asked whether they had noticed a change in women's responses to recommendations for induction in relation to gestational age in light of the pandemic. Around a quarter (24%) said yes. The midwives and doctors reported that women were reluctant to have induction. Women were understandably concerned about not being able to have their partner or a birth supporter with them. More women wanted home birth and were therefore keen to avoid induction. But Harkness *et al* (2021) found that, while women were more likely to want to labour and/or birth at home, *"…the shift to outpatient IOL was clinician-driven rather than service user-driven."*

Both Harkness *et al*'s (2021) study and the outcry that followed the publication of the draft NICE (2021a) guidance highlight that women's experiences, beliefs, knowledge and concerns are not being taken into account.

We need to listen to women.

Women's experiences of induction

There are, of course, many different experiences of labour induction, and some women have very positive experiences. If you search for 'positive induction' or #positiveinduction, you will find lots of stories of women and families who had good experiences. My friend Natalie, for instance, who was probably just about ready to give birth anyway. The tiniest amount of the drug that ripens a woman's cervix sent her into full-blown labour, and she was still able to give birth in the birth centre attached to her local hospital. For her and many others, having labour induced was the right decision.

But it's not a positive experience for everybody. As you will have read in previous sections of this book, some women have very negative experiences of induction which affect them for months, years and, in some cases, decades. Some of the women whose words I have already quoted talked about *being frightened*, having *the worst birth experience* and *feeling traumatised*. These are just samples; I could fill another book with similar quotes. Studies from Sweden (Hildingssen *et al* 2011), Germany (Schwartz *et al* 2016), Australia (Coates *et al* 2019), France (Dupont *et al* 2020) and Finland (Adler *et al* 2020) all confirm that women who experience induction of labour have a higher chance of a negative birth experience. Common themes in the studies are dissatisfaction, lack of information about what induction was going to be like and the fact that induction leads to unwanted interventions and separation from family members.

In 2013, researchers in the UK surveyed 5333 women, of

whom 20% had their labour induced. They found that:

"…*women who were induced were generally less satisfied with aspects of their care and significantly less likely to have a normal delivery. In the qualitative analysis the main themes that emerged concerned delay, staff shortages, neglect, pain and anxiety in relation to getting the induction started and once it was underway; and in relation to failed induction, the main themes were plans not being followed, wasted effort and pain, and feeling let down and disappointed.*" (Henderson & Redshaw 2013: 1159).

A recent Australian study of women's views showed that induction, "…*is a challenging experience for women, which can be understood in terms of the gap between women's needs and the reality of their experience concerning information and decision-making, support, and environment.*" (Coates *et al* 2019).

In a study of women who had been booked for induction at one of eight Sydney hospitals:

"*Most respondents (72%) had hoped to labour spontaneously. Major findings included 19% of women not feeling like they had a choice about induction of labour, 26% not feeling adequately informed (or uncertain if informed), 17% not being given alternatives, and 30% not receiving any written information on induction of labour.*" (Coates *et al* 2020a).

A landmark US project, '*Listening to Mothers,*' is a series of surveys of women's childbearing experiences. The authors identified high levels of induction and other interventions in the first survey (Sakala *et al* 2002). Later reports showed that medicalised birth negatively impacts on women's satisfaction with their birth experience (Declerq *et al* 2007, 2014).

This was also the overall finding of a systematic review on this topic (Lou *et al* 2019). The authors again confirmed that some women are satisfied with their induction experience while others are dissatisfied.

"*Whereas there is substantial and ongoing scientific research on the potential medical advantages and limitations of postterm induction, less is known about the perspectives of the pregnant women. Furthermore, the results of the few existing studies are ambiguous. In a randomized, controlled trial of IOL versus expect-ant care,* [it was] *found that at 41 gestational weeks, 74% of the pregnant women preferred to be induced. In the IOL group, the majority (85%) of induced women reported a positive labor induction experience and 74% would prefer the same management in future pregnancies. However, other studies have found that IOL was associated with less satisfaction, a less-positive birthing experience, and a higher concern for the baby's safety. In an online survey among women with induced labor (all indications), the majority (57%) would not choose IOL in a future pregnancy and requested more information on alternatives and more participation in decision making. These results are important because a negative birth experience is associated with postpartum mental health problems."* (Lou *et al* 2019).

One size clearly doesn't fit all, and we need to take that into account.

Why do some women dislike induction so much?

Several themes are common to almost every study which has looked at why women dislike induction or are dissatisfied after experiencing it. The first is that many women do not feel they were given adequate information about induction beforehand to enable them to be sure that this was right for them (Akuamoah-Boateng & Spencer 2018, Dupont *et al* 2020, Adler *et al* 2020). After they have experienced the reality of an induced labour, they feel they would have made a different decision if they had been properly informed in the first place.

As Akuamoah-Boateng & Spencer (2018) note:

"Unfortunately, the communication of information on IOL has been centered on the risk of prolonged pregnancy without recourse to the risks of the intervention itself making decision about IOL risk averse (Cheyne *et al* 2012)."

The risk averse stance of the medical model, which I discussed in chapter two, may be one reason why so many women report,

"…not feeling that they had a choice about IOL, not being presented with the risks and benefits of different birth options, and receiving insufficient information about the IOL process and

methods." (Coates *et al* 2021: 489).

This is a key issue. The documents and information given to women about induction do tend to gloss over the reality of what it involves, what it is like and what the downsides are. Lou *et al*'s (2019) systematic review also found that:

"…many women experienced IOL to be a 'nondecision.' For example, one woman described how she felt unable to intervene in the IOL protocol or request anything other than what the medical staff suggested. [She said] *Despite being assertive generally, I felt that medical decisions and decisions being made by medical professionals are somehow outside my control."* (Lou *et al* 2019).

Some of the studies looking at women's experiences of induction can help us better understand which aspects of induction are problematic and what could help those women who really need induction for medical reasons. Brown and Furber (2015) carried out research looking at women's experiences of the early stages of the induction process. In this case, the women were on antenatal wards having pessaries inserted into their vaginas to try to make their cervix ripe and ready for birth, which is often the first stage of induction. The hospital was in Wales, and the findings further illustrate why some women dislike induction:

"Strict adherence to ward rules and procedures appeared to undermine women's experiences of cervical ripening as inpatients on an antenatal ward." (Brown & Furber 2015).

Delays were another thing women were frustrated by. Many *"…experienced delays and long waits between admission and the actual induction…"* (Lou *et al* 2019). Visitor restriction has long been an issue; some women were not told that they might spend three or more days on a ward where their partner could only visit during limited hospital visiting times.

"[O]ther examples of the lack of information included cases where women were expected to stay at the hospital, but had not been informed in advance and/or cases where the partner was not allowed to stay overnight at the prenatal ward." (Lou *et al* 2019).

As above, the problem of visitor restriction and personal freedom became far worse during the pandemic, and this was a source of stress and distress for many women and families (Harkness *et al* 2021). Women also reported feeling neglected during the induction process and did not have continuity of carer (Lou *et al* 2019). Many of these issues were raised in a study by Adler *et al* (2020), who found that:

"Overall, 30% of the nulliparous women [those having their first baby] *were dissatisfied (n=231/770) and 19.7% (n=130/659) of the parous women. The specific independent determinants of dissatisfaction for nulliparous women were antenatal birth classes that failed to include discussion of IoL and lack of involvement in the decision-making process. For the parous women, a specific determinant was a delivery that lasted more than 24 hours. Determinants of maternal dissatisfaction common to both groups were unbearable vaginal discomfort, inadequate pain relief, lack of attention to requests, caesarean delivery and severe maternal complications."* (Adler *et al* 2020).

Once we know that there are women who are dissatisfied or traumatised after induction and why they feel this way, the question becomes what we can and should do about this?

Brown and Furber (2015) suggested that:

"Facilitating the continued presence of family members, improving the provision of information, listening to women and enhancing their perception of freedom within the ward environment are strategies that may have a positive influence on women's experiences of inpatient cervical ripening." (Brown & Furber 2015).

I will return to this question. First, I want to add in the experiences of another important group of people, most of whom are also women. The midwives and birth workers who care for those whose labours are being induced. Their perspective can also help us understand the issue.

What do midwives and birth workers think?

During my PhD research, I asked midwives for their knowledge, views and experiences of post-term pregnancy. Often, they expressed deep concern about what happened to women during the process of induction. Here's what midwife

Kate had to say about the unexpected and unwanted physical consequences of induction:

"I just see the morbidity that's attached to that [induction] *and it breaks my heart. All those primips with their syntocinon drip in one arm and their sore fannies from all the prodding and they're on the monitor 'cause there's that whole package that goes with it ... it breaks my heart, and it's flawed, it's fundamentally flawed."* (Kate).

When Kate says, *'it's flawed,'* she is talking about the evidence base for induction. Like many of the midwives and birth workers that I have talked to over the years, she is concerned about two related things. One is the way that induction affects women's experiences. The other, as she describes here, is how recommendations about induction are often made on a relatively arbitrary basis:

"I really have sat in labour wards where it's been a joke, you know, where it's just like it says [in the notes that the woman's due date is] *the 3rd and the 10th and the 17th* [and the staff say] *oh we'll take the 17th, or the 10th, or, with no heed to this incredible thing that's gonna happen to a woman if she gets induced or if we get this date wrong. And nobody seems to care about that, so when these poor lovely women get themselves to term plus ten, nobody really cares whether it's right or wrong. If that's what's filled in the little box or in the notes* [then] *they get induced. And to me, you know, in terms of the oppression, exploitation of women, I mean, I'm so glad you're doing your PhD on induction, 'cause I think it is one of the big central cock-ups of modern medicine, modern maternity care, isn't it?"* (Kate).

One only needs to spend a few minutes reading discussions of unnecessary inductions online to see that many midwives, birth workers and birth activists share Kate's experiences. Some post their stories as blog posts for others to see, and a great example is one written by consultant midwife Helen Shallow, about a woman who was told that her labour needed to be induced because her baby was overdue:

"Lucy was summoned for admission on the Sunday evening, several days after she was advised to be admitted for induction. Her waters were broken in the middle of the night and after two hours the syntocinon drip was commenced; in the early hours of the

morning. Lucy was already exhausted; she had had no sleep for days and no decent nutrition. Eventually she succumbed to an epidural and [her friend] *Fiona described how she only just managed to birth her baby before the team planned further interventions. All this to effect the birth of an allegedly overdue baby."* (Shallow 2019).

Helen goes on to post a picture of the baby (which you can see if you follow the link in the references), inviting colleagues to decide for themselves whether the baby was actually overdue. She adds, *"This little girl was NOT ready to be born, as we can plainly see, by the thick coat of vernix still covering her body. Whereas these are joyful photos for Lucy to treasure, what I see is a baby plucked untimely from the womb."* (Shallow 2019).

The pain and dissonance experienced by those caring for the women having unnecessary inductions, who are often subject to misinformation, unwanted interference (including many vaginal examinations, which many women find embarrassing, uncomfortable and/or distressing), separation from loved ones and iatrogenic pain and complications, is plain to see. In the next section, Heather describes her experience of working as an induction midwife and feeling uncertain about what she can best do to help in this situation. And Anne shared her story of supporting asylum-seeking women, who she says almost always end up having unnecessary inductions:

"I've been involved in the births of 12 asylum-seeking women from different parts of the world, over the past three years, volunteering for a small charity. I have become more and more distressed at the high level of intervention to the point where I don't want to attend another induced birth. Most of our women want and expect a straightforward birth and intend to breast feed. Despite this I have not attended one totally straightforward birth.

The women we accompany generally have had no antenatal care at the point we meet them, and no confirmed due date. So although they are largely young and healthy they are also often Black or Brown and considered high risk. Some of the women have been trafficked. Women who strongly state their needs are overruled, not because the midwives are uncaring, far from it, but the interventions require more investigations and alter the course of the birth. It is a result of a fragmented system where individual needs are subsumed by the needs of the organisation. Many times I have left the hospital in tears because I have been so saddened by what I have seen, as much for the midwives doing their best as for the women whose care isn't good enough." (Anne).

What should we do about it?

Not all researchers agree on what we should do about the fact that so many women are dissatisfied, unhappy and even traumatised after induction of labour. One reason for that is that there are actually two problems that we need to solve. The first is that we clearly need to make the experience of induction better for those women who need it for medical reasons. But we also need to address the issue of unnecessary inductions.

Coates *et al* (2019) call for *"compassionate support"* for those who genuinely need induction. But this is very difficult to implement when health services around the world are being run as businesses (Kirkham 2019).

Henderson and Redshaw (2013) suggested that there was a need for *"...a focused service for these women* [undergoing induction] *to address their additional needs."* Some hospitals have created specific induction services, so that those going into hospital for induction are cared for in designated areas by specialist midwives and other care workers. This can be positive for those women when it is done well. I have met midwives who work in such areas and they are giving care as best they can. But they report that it hasn't solved all of the problems. The inadequacy of information given in pregnancy is still a huge issue. The specialist midwives don't usually get to see women and families until after the decision to induce has been made, at which point they can face a difficult dilemma, as midwife Heather explains.

"They [the women/family] *turn up, and after five minutes it's clear that they've not made an informed decision. They don't really want to be here, they don't really want to be induced and yet what*

can I do at that point? Yes, I can give information and question them, but how far do I go with that, and is it fair? Some have really psyched themselves up for it, and I worry that I might make things worse by introducing doubt at that point. Some might go home, I suppose, and some might just be really confused. More often than not, they are there because someone has told them their baby is at high risk. And we all know that's not true, but I can't guarantee that their baby will be okay if they go home, and that's not because going home is dangerous per se, it's because there are no guarantees. There are no guarantees with induction either. And then, if I talk to them and if they then change their minds and go home, that's going to have to be recorded and I'll be hauled up and have to answer to why, and then the chances are I'm not there to try and make it better for the next family. I'm stuck between a rock and a hard place." (Heather).

There have also been moves in some areas to improve the induction experience by sending women home after giving a cervical ripening agent or inserting a balloon catheter and 'allowing' birth on a midwifery-led unit if women go into labour after this intervention alone. This is sometimes called outpatient induction.

Early research on this is conflicting. One study showed that, *"…women were positive about experiencing the early stages of induction of labour at home with the balloon catheter"* (Coates *et al* 2021). But other research shows that women do not like outpatient induction. Haavisto *et al* (2021) found that, *"…women in the OP* [outpatient] *setting were less satisfied and more anxious than were the women in the IP* [hospital] *setting."*

With this sort of research, we do need to be careful to consider who is being asked and what is being compared, as this can sometimes explain these differences. For instance, Coates *et al* (2021) recruited women who were keen to avoid being given drugs to ripen their cervix, and it is likely that the women in their research were keen to have the balloon catheter method of induction. This may explain why they were so positive about it. I mention this not to detract from the project or the study, but as a reminder that we need to look beyond the findings of studies and consider whether the way they were carried out or the intention behind the study may partly explain why the results are as they are.

It's also important to consider what we're comparing with what. Many areas have already moved towards offering earlier membrane sweeping – which the updated NICE (2021b) guidance also recommends, despite the fact that the 2008 guidance stated that more evidence was needed – and this is often promoted as a way of avoiding 'full blown' induction. Yet we know that women aren't being given good information about this either (Roberts *et al* 2020). And while women may say they prefer membrane sweeping to 'full blown' induction, membrane sweeping is in itself an induction method. Asking women whether they prefer intervention A over intervention B is fine, as long as we remember that we're asking them to compare two medical interventions, and not comparing intervention with awaiting spontaneous labour. If we offered an option C, which was awaiting spontaneous labour in the care of a kind, known midwife who can check that things are okay, answer questions and who you knew would recommend induction if things changed or there was good medical reason to consider it – then some women might prefer that. But when it's not on offer, it's not possible to choose or say you prefer it, so it's important to look at which people and what options were included in the studies.

When I was writing this book, I noticed that the women who were sharing their experiences with me privately were using stronger words (such as *traumatising*, *horrific* and *terrifying*) than are generally seen in research studies. This may be because, as someone who is well known to question induction, I'm more likely to hear from those who feel strongly. Another reason is that women who have had very negative experiences may not want to discuss them with researchers after the fact. Sadly, some women report feeling unable to discuss their feelings with others, especially online, as they are accused of trying to scare other women away from induction. This also happens to those sharing information about induction. It makes the question of how we get accurate information to women and families a really tricky one.

Initiatives such as outpatient induction also don't address the deeper issues. These include the overuse of induction in the first place, the lack or inaccuracy of information given to women and families, the coercive approach that is used by some and the fact that many women's dissatisfaction stems from the fact that their births didn't unfold as they hoped. Many women are more than aware that the journey of birth is unpredictable and doesn't always go to plan. The problem isn't necessarily that women ended up with a different kind of birth from what they had hoped for. It's that they didn't feel that they were able to make decisions themselves. And in some cases women feel that the interventions themselves led to further intervention or health issues, which is why some women feel let down, stressed and/or traumatised when they later realise that they weren't given the full picture before they made the decision to accept induction.

The issue of feeling in control of decision making is not well understood. Dupont *et al* (2020) conclude that, *"…women should be made to feel that they shared in the medical decision to perform IoL."* But such wording implies that the decision is that of the medical professional, whose job it is to make the woman feel as if she participated. In my view, this isn't the answer. One part of the answer is to ensure that women and families actually have unbiased information, and can make their own decision.

This is the view of Lou *et al* (2019) who write that, *"…the experiences of women with induced labor can likely be improved by a communicative and patient-centered approach. To support their informed choice and shared decision making, women need high-quality, unbiased information about IOL, alternative options, and potential outcomes, as well as time to reflect on their personal values and preferences. Women may also need supported opportunities to re-evaluate their hopes and expectations before receiving IOL."*

Their view is shared by those who led the RCM's response

to the draft NICE (2021a) guideline on inducing labour (Brigante & Harley-Lam 2021). It would certainly be a refreshing change from the kind of information that many women and families are currently offered.

Where do we go from here?

I began this chapter by describing how the updated draft NICE (2021a) guideline on inducing labour had caused concern among women, families, midwives, doctors, birth workers and others. I also noted that many individuals and organisations sprang into action to respond to NICE, and that the final version of the guidance (NICE 2021b), which was published in November 2021, had undergone some changes.

While some of the particularly problematic changes and recommendations were removed from the final guideline, other issues remain. The guideline authors removed the suggestion that induction should be offered to certain groups of women, but they did not note that this was not evidence-based. This and a number of other things have been left up to individual Trusts, Health Boards and hospitals. That's worrying, because we know that some groups of women are already being offered induction simply because they are in one of these groups. The NICE guidance includes a statement that variation in practice is problematic and yet when the guidance isn't explicitly clear, variation and what some call the postcode lottery is inevitable.

I noted at the beginning of this chapter that induction will still be offered to healthy, low-risk women, which means that women, families and practitioners need reliable information upon which to base their decisions. My aim in the remainder of this book is to look at some of the situations in which induction is currently offered to healthy, low-risk women, and to explore and explain what the evidence can tell us. I will clarify where there is and is not evidence to help inform decisions, and discuss how it can be vital to look at the quality of that evidence, the wider context and the bigger picture.

4. Due dates, windows and why the computer shouldn't decide

One of my favourite things to post on social media is a picture which points out that the estimated due date is not a 'best before' date, nor a 'give birth by' date. It's a guess. I suggest that, as only 5% of babies are born on their estimated due date, pregnant parents might like to plan to do something nice that day, because they have a 95% chance of being able to keep that appointment.

There is of course always a pedant who points out that you can't have a pedicure or go to the cinema if you give birth two days before your due date.

No, say some of the lovely people who follow me, usually even before I see the reply. They explain that this happened to them, but they kept their date anyway. They had food delivered instead of going out and included their baby in date night. Or they asked the massage therapist to come to their house. Then people start to share the fab and crazy things they planned on their due date or just after. One couple got married the day after their baby's due date, several went on romantic breaks and a personal favourite is the story of the woman who booked a VIP experience on her due date during which she met her favourite actor. He apparently looks slightly terrified in the souvenir photo, presumably at the idea that she might suddenly give birth, but that's another story.

There are many reasons that I love to read the responses to this post. The main one is that it is evidence of a growing understanding that an estimated due date *is* just a guesstimate, and that perhaps we need to resist the power it has been given in recent years.

The fact that due dates aren't accurate is just one part of the problem that they cause, though. In this chapter, I'll look at the history, the research evidence and the issues that stem from our use of due dates, and why it really is time that we looked at other possible approaches.

Where's the problem?

Our culture, for the reasons outlined in chapter two, has fully embraced the idea of due dates. We accept that they are 'a thing' (even though they are totally man made, as I'll discuss in this chapter). We allow due dates to dictate many of our actions, thoughts and conventions around pregnancy. The idea of the due date is often embedded in the very first thing we say when we learn that someone is pregnant – *"Ooooh, congratulations, when are you due?"* It acts as a marker for many of the tests offered in pregnancy. It helps us decide when to order the birth pool, pack the hospital bag and put someone on call to look after siblings. If we lived in a different time and place, due dates might not be as important. In our culture, the due date is a crucial piece of information which helps us organise our lives. So where's the problem?

Well, the estimated due date has a far greater significance than being the deadline for the buying of nappies or making sure the car is filled with petrol. It can create an expectation which isn't accurate, and I've already briefly mentioned that due dates are imprecise. Many readers will be aware that due dates and the expectations that go along with them can lead to family stress and pressure, as I said in the introduction to this book.

Another issue is that they are often assigned by a professional, or even a machine, and the woman's own knowledge may not be taken into account. Many women dislike this, and then get even more fed up with medical professionals changing their due date after a later ultrasound scan, often continuing to ignore their own dates or the fact that they know exactly when they conceived. No sooner has someone got used to one date (though they might still be stressing over the first one, which perhaps didn't take account of their personal circumstances), than some whiz with an ultrasound machine comes along and changes it.

"They said the computer system wouldn't allow them to change it back." (Debbie).

It's concerning that we live in a culture where machines are allowed to override other kinds of knowledge, like the fact that your egg was implanted on your wife's birthday in July, so you couldn't possibly have conceived in August. Or that you really can be certain about when you conceived, because your boyfriend is in the military and had exactly one day's leave in the past eight weeks.

But perhaps the most significant implication of the due date is the induction date that is set, sometimes automatically and without discussion or consent, in an attempt to ensure that women don't stay pregnant for too long after their due date. In some areas and situations, because the due date is generally set at 40 completed weeks of pregnancy and induction is now offered to some women at 39 weeks, induction is offered even before the due date is reached.

There is an assumption that the baby suddenly becomes endangered after a certain arbitrary date if it remains in its mother's womb, as if babies have a 'use by' date like foods do. Many women therefore feel they should go along with an induction no matter what they feel and believe. Assigning a due date, allowing a machine to change it and then using that date to determine the end point of pregnancy sends a very clear message. It conveys the idea than medical science knows more about when a baby should be born than either the baby herself or the woman whose body has created, grown and nourished her baby. Whether an induction date is set early or late in pregnancy, it undermines a woman's ability to birth her baby when the time is right. This is the epitome of the Enlightenment ideal: that men who do science can control nature. But these ideas aren't evidence-based and they can do more harm than good to women and babies.

Our ideas around the due date also suggest that something awful will happen if the baby hasn't arrived by a certain point in pregnancy. As I discussed in chapter three, it can cause immense stress when someone is told that labour needs to be induced because the baby is 'at risk' and then is later told, *'Oh sorry, there's no bed for you til Monday.'* Or they go to hospital on the date they were given – because they're now worried and believe that their body is going to fail after the set date – and find that it takes three days for them to get into labour.

This might all sound a bit stark, but it's important to understand due dates, because so many of us have accepted them without being told how they have come about. Many people feel reassured and better about their own body after reading about the actual history and evidence relating to due dates. Knowledge is power. I'm not going to get to the end of this chapter and suggest we throw out estimated due dates. That wouldn't be helpful, even if it were possible. But once you know a few key things about due dates, and about the research relating to the end of pregnancy (which I cover in the next chapter), you might decide to see due dates differently. You might give them a bit less power. You might take back control from the ultrasound and computer systems and develop more trust in your body and your baby.

Because the crazy thing is that, when you look closely at what we know about the length of pregnancy, you find something rather curious: you find that it isn't based on good evidence. You find, in fact, that it's a bit like a house of cards. If you give the theories one good poke to see what they're made of, the whole thing collapses. In other words, the policy of induction at a certain point in pregnancy is largely based on fear, tradition, fashion and some outdated, misogynistic ideas rather than sound evidence.

Let me explain.

The history of the due date

Some people think that, way back in time, women used the lunar cycle and the seasons to get a sense of when their baby would be born, but we don't know this. Archaeologists have found ancient artifacts such as the notched Lebombo and Ishango animal bones, which appear to be calendars or calculators. In the 1970s, an archaeologist pointed out that these might have been used by women, to chart their own menstrual cycles or fertility (Zaslavsky 1979, 1991). This idea has been picked up by those writing about birth, midwifery and women's cycles (Sjöö & Mor 1991, van der Kooy 1994). But it's only one theory, and there are others, which centre on the bones being evidence of the early origins of maths (Everett 2017, Padmanabhan & Padmanabhan 2019, Born 2021).

We also think that ancient Hindu and Roman cultures had a sense of pregnancy length (Saunders & Paterson 1991). But the earliest written record comes from Aristotle, who lived about 2,400 years ago. He wrote that the average length of pregnancy was ten lunar months, which we have long taken to mean 280 days (van der Kooy 1994, Rosser 2000). But there is a bit of debate about that, too. Aristotle seems to have recorded a cultural belief about pregnancy lasting ten lunar months rather than undertaking systematic observation (van der Kooy 1994). Elverdam and Wielandt (1994) argue that this figure was likely based on ancient cultural preferences for celestially significant numbers such as seven and 40, which multiply to make 280. Whether that's true or not, there's no evidence that Aristotle's guesstimate is based on research. Although, as I will discuss in this chapter, there are a number of reasons why using the same calculation to assign a fixed due date to everyone is problematic, even if it were based on robust research.

The obstetric construct of post-term pregnancy was first written about in 1709. That's when a Dutch doctor, Hermann Boerhaave, proposed an algorithm (or set of rules) which would estimate the date of birth. He did that by adding seven days and nine months to the date of a woman's last menstrual period, or LMP (Speert 1958). Somewhat ironically, given how it impacts us today, there is a suggestion that the measurement of gestational length has legal rather than medical roots. Doctors were called upon to decide whether the time that had elapsed between sex and birth could positively establish paternity (Saunders & Paterson 1991). This shows how women weren't listened to or believed then either. Doctors could override a woman's knowledge and declare whether a particular man might or might not be the father of her baby. As you might imagine, the medical men's pronouncements weren't always truthful, especially if they were bribed by the alleged father. This prioritising of doctors' knowledge over women's knowledge and experiences sadly continues today, still to the detriment of women.

I want to add a note about a word I used in the previous paragraph. We call post-term pregnancy a construct because it's a theory. It's an idea that has been proposed by humans. But ideas aren't automatically true, even if lots of people believe them. Many stereotypes are applied to different groups of people, for instance, and some of them might be widely accepted as true, but that doesn't make them so. The only way we can know whether a construct or theory is true or not is to carry out robust research to test the theory.

The due date is just one of many health and medical constructs or theories which are based on something that someone thought up. Often, the numbers and timeframes are arbitrary. When we trace their roots, we sometimes find that they have a solid basis. But sometimes we find that they were indeed made up. The reason, for example, that we are encouraged to take 10,000 steps a day has nothing to do with this being the optimal number for our health. It's because, when the Japanese company Yamasa Clock invented a step tracker in 1965, they called it the *Manpo-Lei*, which means '10,000 steps meter.' The Japanese character for the number 10,000 looks like a person walking, which cemented this as a marketing device. Many people still use this number as their goal today even though there's no evidence that 10,000 steps is linked with optimal health. In fact, research now shows that about 7000 steps a day is optimal and more steps than that may not add any benefit (Lee *et al* 2019, Paluch *et al* 2021).

But back to due dates. Hermann Boerhaave's algorithm was reported by Franz Carl Naegele and is commonly known as Naegele's rule (Naegele 1830, Speert 1958, van der Kooy 1994). Unfortunately, neither Naegele nor Boerhaave noted whether the length of pregnancy should be estimated from the first or last day of the woman's last menstrual period. Yet the writers of obstetric textbooks decided that it should be the first day. This means that the estimated length of pregnancy used today may be shorter than the originators of this theory intended. Not that their suggestion was based on research in the first place, though.

Over the years, research has shown that Naegele's rule doesn't accurately reflect the average length of pregnancy. A few small, older studies found that the average length of pregnancy was a few days longer than Naegele's rule predicts (Bergjso *et al* 1990, Mittendorf *et al* 1990). A later, larger study (Smith 2001) confirmed that the median average length of pregnancy, or the point by which half of all women had given birth, was 40 weeks and five days. More recently still, Jukic *et al* (2013) collected urine samples from women so they could accurately measure when conception occurred. Their results also showed that the average length of pregnancy was a few days longer than Naegele's rule predicts. As I will discuss in more depth below, this research also found considerable variation in length of pregnancy between women, even when the conception date was known.

The construct of the due date and related constructs such as post-term pregnancy depend on three things. The first is the idea that we can accurately define the average length of pregnancy. The second is that we can use that to create an algorithm which can calculate a standardised due date for everyone. In the next chapter, I'll look at the third one, which is the idea that there is an optimum length of pregnancy. But even a quick look at the evidence debunks the idea that we can accurately measure the average length of pregnancy with a 'one size fits all' approach. The industrial approach of finding standardised ways to measure individuals so you can manage and monitor people through a process – in this case pregnancy and birth – doesn't work here. However, as some of my research participants said (often in rather colourful language), the idea that due dates are accurate and useful has become embedded in our culture. But when you think about it, it's amazing that so many women today are affected by something that was decided rather arbitrarily so long ago and without any research to support it. And even though research has since shown it to be inaccurate, its use has continued.

"OK, so Aristotle says pregnancy is ten lunar months la la la and then that gets carried down through generations and somehow it gets co-opted into the obstetric [deeper voice] *this is how it is. And so all this research is based on this initial assumption made by, oh, some three thousand year old Greek bloke ... And it's nuts, when you think about it. Just nuts."* (Cerridwyn).

"I think, as a society, there's something about us, it's one of our rituals, isn't it? That date. Because that whole shite that women get put through that go past their date, that kind of 'you're failing to conform in some way' and cause a bit of a nuisance ... 'would you hurry up please, you're holding my life up.'" (Sally).

Fixed-point expectation syndrome

A few years ago, I invented a construct of my own. It's called fixed-point expectation syndrome. I decided that, if believers in the technocratic approach to birth can create syndromes and terms to label people and make something sound as if it is worthy of time, attention, analysis and research funding, I could do the same.

Fixed-point expectation syndrome describes a state that we can enter anytime we're looking forward to something. Maybe the arrival of something you've ordered online. News about whether you're going to be offered an exciting new job. Or when you're waiting to see if someone you like messages. We can't help but have an expectation of the date and time on which we think the thing we're anticipating should occur. When it doesn't arrive or happen on time, we may experience negative feelings. We've been let down; maybe even ghosted. Commercial companies capitalise on this by inviting us to pay extra to have our things guaranteed to arrive the next day.

I'm not judging or blaming anyone who can relate to this

feeling, and I'm certainly not going to get too deeply into whether this is right or wrong, but I will note that the pressure we can sometimes feel about time and what needs to happen and when are another consequence of capitalist, technocratic culture. Fixed-point expectation syndrome is a very modern state and, just as with some other aspects of our culture, you can decide whether you want to allow it to be a part of your life or not. The point here is that estimated dates and delivery windows are deemed to be necessary and beneficial in consumer culture, and many of us are used to being able to get things when we want them. Some of us also find it hard to wait for things we really want.

But there's a huge difference between waiting for parcels and waiting for babies. Your parcel, text or job offer may or may not arrive on time, but in most cases it won't have a long-term impact. When it's not a book but a baby, the impact is greater. Magnify the excitement of the parcel by a million, give a delivery estimate that's several months away and then see how much fixed-point expectation follows.

This is exactly what we do when we use a due date to mark when we think birth might happen. But nature can't be predicted or scheduled in the way a product delivery can. That is, unless you induce labour or schedule a caesarean, which might be one reason why the rates of both have gone up even though they carry risks and downsides for women and babies. But even then, the maternity services may need to change the scheduled date if they can't accommodate the original plan, so even that's not a certainty, and there's no money-back guarantee if things don't work out as hoped.

We're all individual. Our bodies and growth patterns vary. Pregnancy length varies, and some babies just need more time than others. Most importantly, there isn't a direct link between average and optimal. When it comes to the timing for birth, there isn't an optimal fixed-point that we can calculate and give to everyone. There isn't just one day on which a baby can be born happily and healthily.

My friend and long-time editor Julie Frohlich is a

consultant midwife who spends a lot of time talking women through their labour and birth options. When it comes to induction for being 'overdue,' she has a favourite phrase (Wickham 2018a). *"Your baby is not going to turn into a pumpkin at midnight,"* she tells women. In reality, absolutely nothing happens at the stroke of midnight on your due date, or on any other date relating to it. The due date is a construct. Normality is a range. And it's important to talk more about that.

Normality is a range

Midwives have long pointed out that it's not helpful to use a fixed-point estimated due date, and many use terms like guess date or guesstimate to communicate this to women and families. As I discussed in chapter one, there is a span of several weeks in which a baby can be optimally born. It's true that being born too early can lead to poorer outcomes. It's also true that being born very late can lead to a slightly higher chance of stillbirth, as I discuss in chapter five. Induction has downsides of its own though, so there's a need to weigh up the pros and cons. But the vast majority of babies, if allowed to decide for themselves when labour should begin, will be born within the span that we have traditionally called term.

In a classic article, midwife Brenda van der Kooy noted that, *"...as elsewhere in nature, normality has a range"* (1994: 5) and called for change in the way we approach due dates. Stickler (1994: 325) also recommended using *"...less specific terminology such as 'month of expected delivery'* ... [which] *would cure the many ills stemming from the pseudoaccuracy of the EDC* [expected date of confinement]." My research found that midwives practising outside of the system (who therefore had more freedom to decide how they worked) used the idea of a wider window (Wickham 2009b, 2011). This more accurately reflected reality and it also removed the problem of fixed-point expectation syndrome for women and families.

"I always talk to them about having a due month, and, you know, if that is like the beginning to the end of a month or [from]

the middle of a month to the next." (Xena).

"[I tell women] *a lot that the date is not a set date, that it's actually a whole month that the baby can be born in. If* [the estimated due date is] *June 16th she should be ready between the 1st and the 30th of June, anytime."* (Anna Andhra)

The interesting thing about Naegele's rule is that, while it's only accurate for one in 20 women if you focus on the date it points to, it isn't bad at predicting when a baby will be born if we use it as the central point of a range of time. A study from 1967 (which in this case is useful, because fewer women were having their labours induced back then) showed that 70% of all live births occurred within 280 ± 10 days of each woman's LMP (Treloar *et al* 1967a). The "± 10 days" bit means that 70% of the babies were both in a 21-day period which spanned from ten days before the due date to ten days after the due date. This is exactly what the midwives in my research meant by a wider window. They generally talked about a four-week window rather than Treloar *et al*'s (1967a) three week one.

But it's also important to remember that 30% of the babies in Treloar *et al*'s (1967a) study weren't born within that three-week window, and most were healthy. This is the challenge when we use an average or standard. We need to ensure that in assuring a percentage of the population that it is 'normal,' we don't leave out a smaller but significant number of people who are also healthy and 'normal' even if their experience falls a bit outside the boundaries set by things like due dates and guidelines. Remember, the boundaries are constructs; they're not always based on evidence, and we're all different.

There is evidence that women prefer a wider window approach too. This was certainly the experience of the midwives in my research (Wickham 2009b, 2011). And in a survey of 769 women in Sydney, Australia, most understood that the expected date of birth was imprecise. Most of the women wished that the estimated timing of their birth could be given in less specific format than a single due date, with the majority preferring the idea of an estimated week or fortnight of birth (Todd *et al* 2017).

Why the variation?

I mentioned that research has shown that a number of factors can influence the length of pregnancy. These factors include the length of a woman's menstrual cycle, her age and educational level (Treloar *et al* 1967a, Jukic *et al* 2013, Oberg *et al* 2013). Genetic variations, ancestry and the length of a woman's mother's and grandmother's pregnancies may also play a part (Mittendorf 1990, 1993, Mogren *et al* 1999, Morken *et al* 2011, Oberg *et al* 2013, Lawson 2021). The baby's father's genes influence pregnancy length too (Lie *et al* 2006), and maternal weight (Jukic *et al* 2013, Oberg *et al* 2013), height (Mittendorf 1990, 1993, Chan & Lao 2009, Derraik *et al* 2016) and diet (McAlpine *et al* 2016) can also lead to variation. We know that, in women who have already had a baby, the length of later pregnancies is related to the length of their previous pregnancies (Ng & Steer 2016). In other words, shorter-than-average and longer-than-average pregnancies tend to recur. Out of interest, this sort of variation doesn't only exist in relation to the length of pregnancy. We also know from recent research that there is a strong positive association between mother and daughter lengths of labour (Ebrahimoff *et al* 2020). But we have no idea why this is the case.

Not only is there variation in the length of different women's menstrual cycles (Treloar *et al* 1967b, Jukic *et al* 2013), but also when they ovulate. We know that menstrual cycle length doesn't just vary between women; it also varies over a woman's reproductive lifetime. And not everyone remembers the date of their LMP, especially if they weren't planning to become pregnant. Variation is healthy and normal. Variation exists because, with a few exceptions, birth works best when babies get to decide when they are ready to be born. But this variation isn't being taken into account in standardised guidelines, which assume that 'one size fits all.'

Every few years, an obstetrician will write about this in a medical journal, pointing out that the metaphorical emperor is naked. One of the most recent is Lawson (2021), who wrote in the Australian and New Zealand Journal of Obstetrics and Gynaecology that:

"...what might have been an appropriate formula in Germany in the 19th century deserves to be revisited in the 21st ... Naegele's rule should be considered as a guideline for the expected date of confinement, and not a definite date." Lawson (2021: 177).

Like others before him, his article was ignored by his colleagues, who carried on doing what they've always done.

Is ultrasound more accurate?

Women and families are often told that ultrasound is a more accurate way of estimating the due date than using Naegele's rule and a woman's LMP date. People often cite a Cochrane review by Whitworth *et al* (2015) in support of the accuracy of ultrasound due dates. But the authors of that review note that the evidence is of low quality and the findings aren't as robust as some of those who quote the review imply. It no longer appears on the list of current Cochrane reviews. That said, some smaller and good quality studies have found ultrasound to be more accurate than LMP dates (Jukic *et al* 2013). But there's a catch. This statement is only true on a population basis. That's because, as I've already explained, Naegele's rule is a fairly blunt instrument and there are several potential points where error or uncertainty can enter the equation. A proportion of women will still have an inaccurate due date if it is calculated by ultrasound. Partly because 'normal' is a range and nature exhibits variation. I apologise for the repetition, but it really does come back to this every time.

Due dates generated by ultrasound use an entirely different principle from Naegele's rule and the LMP date. Ultrasound dating of pregnancy is based on the theory that there is a link between the size of the baby and the length of pregnancy. And there is a link in a crude sense, of course. A 12-week-old fetus is nowhere near the size of a baby born at 36 weeks. When we're looking at the difference of a week or two, though, things get trickier. So what have researchers discovered about the accuracy of ultrasound dating?

Khambalia *et al*'s (2013) study analysed data from 18,708 women who went into spontaneous labour between 2007 and 2011 in Australia. They compared the estimated and actual date of birth for each woman/baby. It's important to remember that studies which look at data in this way are only as good as the medical records that were kept at the time, but we don't have better data on this particular question.

They found (as I've already stated) that only 5% of babies were born on their due date and that about 66% of births occurred within seven days either side of the estimated date of birth. This does make ultrasound a bit more accurate at predicting the date of birth on a population basis than the use of Naegele's rule and a woman's LMP date. Remember that, with LMP dates, 70% of babies are born within ten days either side of their LMP due date, so the difference isn't huge.

There is also an important caveat. As I noted above, if something is accurate for the 66% or 70% of women whose babies are born in the predicted window, that's great for them. We can't know who they are until afterwards, of course, but we can say that about seven out of ten women get a due date which predicts the date of their baby's birth within a two- or three-week period. But it's not so great for the 30-34% of healthy women who go into spontaneous labour at term whose pregnancy will be longer or shorter than that. That's about one in three women.

One reason for ultrasound dating being inaccurate for about a third of women is because there is variation in the growth of babies in utero. This shouldn't surprise us. There is variation in the growth and size of two-month-olds, five-year-olds and seventeen-year-olds. And during a woman's pregnancy, when you're measuring tiny distances on a screen that's projecting an image picked up by ultrasound waves travelling through her body, you're not always going to get it right. This is no criticism of sonographers. It's just that technology is limited, and machines aren't infallible.

The fact that normal growth is a range that can lead to errors in estimation was confirmed by a Swedish study. Researchers looked at the growth of babies in utero who had been conceived by IVF, so they would know exactly when conception took place. They measured the babies by ultrasound at different stages of pregnancy so they could see if the ultrasound estimates of their age accurately reflected their actual age (Källén *et al* 2013). For the most part, the ultrasound estimates of the baby's age matched with their actual age. But there wasn't a good match in every case. For some women there is more likelihood of an error if ultrasound is used to predict a due date. The researchers found that:

"In most IVF pregnancies, routine fetometry [or measuring babies by ultrasound] *correctly predicts gestational age but deviations exist which indicate that ultrasound underestimates the age of fetuses that will be born small for gestational age and when the woman is obese."* (Källén *et al* 2013: 372).

Kullinger *et al* (2016) also found that some groups of women are more likely to be affected by ultrasound dating errors. Their research showed us who is more likely to have their due date changed to an earlier date by ultrasound (because their baby is bigger than the LMP date suggests it should be). Some are more likely to have their due date put back to a later date because the baby is smaller than expected.

The women most likely to have their due date made earlier because their baby was larger than expected were those with a body mass index (BMI) of 40 kg/m^2 or higher. But larger women aren't alone in being affected by this.

"Other factors associated with large negative discrepancies were: diabetes, young maternal age, multiparity, body mass index between 30 and 39.9 kg/m^2 or <18.5 kg/m^2, a history of gestational diabetes, female fetus, shorter stature (<−1 SD), a history of pre-eclampsia, smoking or snuff use, and unemployment." (Kullinger *et al* 2016)

Women in this situation can end up being advised to have their labour induced at a time when, by their own calculations, they aren't as pregnant as the computer system now says they are. I hear from many women in this situation. They are often distressed, because they have been told that their baby may be in danger if they don't accept induction, yet they are sure that their baby isn't ready to be born.

Some women also had large positive discrepancies in Kullinger *et al*'s (2016) research, where the baby was a boy, where the woman was over 30, had given birth before or was taller. These are the women who, having had a due date calculated from their LMP, are told that their expected date of delivery will be changed to a later date. This can also be distressing, because women may want their labour induced if for instance they go beyond 41 weeks but, if their due date is made later, induction may not be offered at the correct time.

In total, Kullinger *et al*'s (2016) study showed that more than one in six women were found to have a due date discrepancy of more than a week when an ultrasound date is calculated after an LMP date has been assigned. Some women had a discrepancy of 20 days.

Before I move away from discussing ultrasound dating, I also want to mention that due date changes after a scan can happen in late pregnancy in some areas. This is in spite of the fact that there is far greater variation in the size of babies in late pregnancy and there is no evidence that late ultrasound due date estimation is accurate. In fact, the increasing variation in the size of babies that inevitably occurs as pregnancy progresses means that it is likely to be increasingly inaccurate (Bricker *et al* 2015).

Dating approaches and individualised care

It's very clear from the research that, if a woman isn't sure of her LMP dates, an ultrasound scan is likely to be the most accurate means of estimating a due date. But if the woman is confident in her LMP date, there is no evidence that an ultrasound due date is preferable:

"On a population basis, there were no meaningful differences in the prediction of date of birth by ultrasound scan date. An early

dating scan (≤ 10 weeks) is unnecessary if LMP is reliable." (Khambalia *et al* 2013).

However, some people recommend that, where there is a discrepancy, the ultrasound date is used in preference to a woman's own LMP date (Lawson 2021). As I have already noted, this can cause immense frustration and distress to some women. Women often report that the new date is imposed on them in an authoritarian way rather than treated as a guesstimate. Just as when due dates were created so that doctors could make pronouncements about paternity, the advent of ultrasound dating has meant that the woman herself doesn't generally get a say. Instead, as we've seen, the date is changed, sometimes automatically by a computer system, as the result of the findings of a machine, or on the say so of a person she may have never met before.

The underlying but inaccurate message is the same: *we know more about your pregnancy than you do*. The problem, again, is that maternity services tend to take a one size fits all approach. That's how bureaucracies are run.

The due date is an intervention

In summarising the issues in this chapter, perhaps the most important thing that I can say about the construct of the estimated due date is that it is an intervention. But unlike many birth interventions – which include screening tests, preventative measures, and drugs and procedures intended to treat specific conditions – we don't tend to think of it as such. We're so used to having due dates that we don't think of them in the same way as, say, episiotomies or oxytocin drips. But the estimated due date is a means of measuring pregnancy so that it can then be managed.

As I've shown in this chapter, women aren't asked if they want a due date estimated. There's no informed choice here. In fact, the idea that the due date is a key part of being pregnant is so ingrained in most of us that we have worked one out for ourselves even before we see a midwife or doctor.

Most women aren't given information about the uncertainty or risks associated with pregnancy dating or any choice in how their estimated due date is calculated by those working in systems of maternity care. Unless they opt out of ultrasound scans (which some women do; nothing is compulsory), there's always the possibility that the date will be changed without the woman's consent and sometimes against her will. This is both extraordinary and worrying given that, as I'll discuss further in chapter five, the due date is an intervention which can significantly impact a woman's experience and decision making.

That said, I'm not arguing that we do away with due dates. What I am suggesting is that we widen our thinking and make estimated due dates part of a conversation rather than an assumption. Due dates are an intervention, they aren't really that accurate and we shouldn't be allowing one of the most important and impactful pregnancy interventions to be set and changed by a computer without the woman's consent.

In the next chapter, I'll continue this conversation by discussing the issues that arise when the length of a pregnancy progresses beyond the estimated due date and into the related construct of 'post-term' pregnancy.

5. Induction in late pregnancy – your baby isn't like a pumpkin

"I am so confused."

I looked up at Eddie, a medical student who I was tutoring in research methods. He was clutching my 'Inducing Labour: making informed decisions' (Wickham 2018a) book in one hand and a copy of a research paper (I think the ARRIVE Trial, and we'll come to that) in the other. He waved them around a bit, for emphasis. *"It's like there are two totally different worlds here. Speaking different languages."*

"There kind of are," I replied, nodding. *"It's hard to make sense of, I know."*

"And as far as I can tell," he continued, as he sat down and pulled a notebook out of his bag, *"it boils down to what you believe."*

"You're right," I agreed. *"And whether your priority is the numbers, the money and the short-term outcomes, even if the benefits are really marginal, or the wider picture of women and families and the potential impact on longer term health and wellbeing."*

He sighed. *"We should change the relationship status of the induction research to, 'it's complicated',"* he said, and I laughed. Many a true word has been spoken in jest.

A tiny bit more history

Just like the due date, the notion of post-term pregnancy is a construct. It's just over a hundred years old, and someone made it up. This concept doesn't exist in nature, and vets don't go around inducing animal's births just because pregnancy has 'gone on too long.'

The first modern reference to post-term pregnancy is widely credited to Ballantyne (1902). He wrote about how a few babies were born with a 'wasting' condition. They were slimmer than other babies and, although they perked up after a few good feeds, they didn't initially appear as healthy. Several decades passed and then a German obstetrician, Runge, theorised that this condition, *"...might be due to impairment of the nutrient supply line to the fetus."* (Oakley 1984: 177). In other words, there may be a problem with the placenta.

This seems to be the first suggestion from modern medicine that placentas could be 'insufficient,' which means that they might fail to deliver the nutrients the baby needs. And, in fact, it is a correct suggestion in that a few women and babies do experience placental insufficiency. But placental insufficiency only occurs occasionally and affects a very small number of people. However, this initial observation of an occasional problem has, over the years, grown into the unscientific idea that every placenta is always on the brink of failing, especially in later pregnancy. This myth now forms part of the justification for routinely interfering with the end of pregnancy.

Again, as we saw with the construct of the due date in the last chapter, the placental insufficiency theory implies that pregnancy has a 'best before' date. In fact, placentas can begin to work less efficiently at any point in pregnancy, but they generally do a marvellous job. Genuine insufficiency is unusual, but it happens occasionally. There is no evidence that placentas routinely fail once they reach a certain age, and it doesn't tend to happen overnight.

"As an obstetrician friend of mine likes to say, if a woman's placenta isn't working well at 23 weeks, then it is unlikely to be working well by 39 weeks. But if it is working well at 40 or 41 weeks then there's no good reason to think its function is suddenly going to decline over the next few days." (Wickham 2018a: 58).

For all these reasons, it's better to monitor the health and wellbeing of each individual woman and baby and to remember that everyone is different, rather than relying on unproven assumptions which mean we intervene too soon in some cases and not soon enough in others. Yet some people believe in and promote the unproven and unhelpful idea that, once we pass our due date, our bodies start to fail our babies.

The second bit of history that I want to share is to do with how methods of inducing labour became the domain of medicine. Hot, tired, fed-up-of-still-being-pregnant women have likely been trying ways of encouraging their bodies to get on and have their babies for a long time, but this was a personal thing. Methods of induction were discussed in the textbooks published after the Enlightenment era, when obstetrics started to become a good way to earn a living (Murphy-Lawless 1998). This era also saw moves to discredit midwives, who had always supported women and families in birth. Knowledgeable, independent women (and that's what midwives often were, for families would pay them in kind, which meant they didn't need to rely on a man for support) are threatening to the establishment. Attempts to undermine and discredit midwives continue today, despite evidence that midwifery care leads to the best outcomes for healthy women and babies (Sandall *et al* 2016).

From the 1950s, doctors began to suggest that babies were at risk if they remained in the womb for too long (Clifford 1954), and two research studies claimed to link prolonged pregnancy with a higher chance of neonatal death (Hasseljo & Auberg 1962, Lanman 1968). Now considered to be poorly designed, these studies aren't included in current reviews. But the myth I described in chapter two had taken hold. People began to distrust that, on the whole, women's and babies' bodies were the best determinant of when labour should begin. They believed the new idea that, if pregnancy continued for too long, babies were in danger in the womb.

The final step in the 1960s was *"a reliable infusion system for oxytocin-based drugs"* (Murphy-Lawless 1998: 202). In other words, that's when it became possible to give manufactured oxytocin through an intravenous drip. Once a product to help induce or accelerate labour appeared, induction rates started to rise. As Ann Oakley wrote, *"The era of the womb's sanctity as a private, peaceful place is, indeed, over."* (Oakley 1984: 180).

Why it's complicated

There's a lot of disagreement about post-term pregnancy and the value of routinely offering induction towards the end of pregnancy. That's partly because many of the individual studies show no difference in the stillbirth rate between induction and expectant management. We use the term 'expectant management,' to mean waiting for labour to begin on its own; checking that the woman and baby are okay and offering intervention only in situations where there is a genuine reason, rather than just a risk factor. Expectant management means that induction is still offered in case of a medical condition or other problem being detected. Some midwives call this 'watchful waiting.'

We do know that there is a slight increase in rates of stillbirth once pregnancy continues past a certain point. But the increase occurs later than many people think and is also less than most people think. Researchers and reviews disagree about whether induction of labour prevents stillbirth or leads to better outcomes overall (Wickham 2018a, Seijmonsbergen-Schermers *et al* 2020). It's possible that induction saves some babies but it may harm others, because the powerful drugs used can cause fetal distress and lead to more interventions which also have side effects.

The studies cited in favour of routine induction for post-term pregnancy only look at short-term physical outcomes. They don't consider things like mental health or the medium- and long-term consequences of induction (Seijmonsbergen-Schermers *et al* 2019, 2020, Dahlen *et al* 2021), which I discussed in chapter one. So even if induction confers a small reduction in stillbirth, it leads to *"...higher birth interventions, particularly in primiparous women, and more adverse maternal, neonatal and child outcomes."* (Dahlen *et al* 2021).

It's also important to know that sadly, stillbirth sometimes occurs even when there are no risk factors. Up to a third of stillbirths that happen in pregnancy have no known cause (Warland & Mitchell 2014).

There's one more important issue when it comes to the induction research. Like the early medical men who sought to take business from midwives, some people profit from promoting induction. Some of those I cite in this chapter have financial or other interests in pharmaceutical companies who manufacture and sell induction drugs. For others, the promotion of induction brings research funding, job security, and prestige. If you look at any of the papers that I am citing, or at other health- or birth-related research, have a look at the 'competing interests' section. It's fascinating to see how often studies promoting drugs or interventions are written by those who directly and personally profit from their use.

The actual risk of stillbirth

When it comes to discussing risk in relation to the chance of stillbirth at the end of pregnancy, this quote summarises what the Royal College of Midwives (RCM) in the UK deems best practice for professional midwives, and formed part of their response to the 2021 draft NICE guidance, which did not take a woman-centred approach. It's deemed important to tell women that the research findings are uncertain, and to describe the chance of stillbirth in numbers.

"Women should be informed that the body of evidence on the gestational age beyond which continuing the pregnancy may pose any additional risks to mother and/or baby is contradictory. That said, there is some evidence that although small, the risk of stillbirth or perinatal death in the first week of life may increase with expectant management between 41 and 42 weeks, roughly from less than one per 1000 pregnancies to four per 1000. We should provide this information to women in clear absolute risk terms, developing infographics from the body of research evidence and enable women to decide what's best for them in their individual circumstances. We should not just refer to 'increased risk' and make decisions for them … we should provide women with the information and evidence based on their personal circumstances including risk, so that they can make an informed decision." (Brigante & Harlev-Lam 2021).

Unfortunately, as this quote from my mailbox shows, this ideal isn't always reflected in reality. Although not everyone feels as strongly as Yasmin about the way that information was given to her, many women and families describe similar experiences to hers.

"She [the obstetric registrar] *told me that, if I didn't agree to be induced, my baby was four times more likely to die, and was I really wanting to take that risk, because it was on my head and not hers if I did. Of course I said yes. Later, I found out the actual numbers. I'll never forgive that woman for the way she manipulated the statistics to persuade me to do what she wanted."* (Yasmin).

There is a really important difference between giving someone information in relative terms – for instance, saying that you're twice as likely to have X, or three times as likely to experience Y – and in absolute terms, by sharing the actual numbers. Most people recommend that risks and benefits are discussed in absolute terms. As Brigante and Harlev-Lam (2021) and consultant midwives like Julie Frohlich (personal correspondence 2018) recommend, infographics can help show what these risks really look like, for instance by sharing a picture showing one woman in a thousand. Our brains find it easier to make sense of this kind of information.

The statistics on stillbirth at the end of pregnancy vary with every study. That's partly because researchers don't all agree on how we should measure this. For a start, they don't agree on who we should compare with who. Measuring the number of babies born in a single week is the easy part, though the accuracy of this depends on the accuracy of due dates. Which, as we know from chapter four, aren't very accurate. Over the years, the way we calculate stillbirth rates by week of pregnancy has changed. There are now two or three different ways to calculate stillbirth risk, and not everybody agrees which is best. In fact, there may be no 'best' way, because there are too many uncertainties and human factors involved.

But that's just one reason why there is variation in the studies. Another reason for variation is that studies include different kinds of women experiencing different kinds of maternity care, depending on when and where the study was conducted. Nowadays, we are probably saving some babies who would have died in earlier years, which is why it can be unhelpful and misleading to use older research studies. On the other hand, more babies are being exposed to the harms of induction and other interventions, and these can sometimes be the cause of illness, stillbirth or perinatal death. So for all of these reasons and more, we just can't be completely accurate here.

That said, there are some things that we can be confident about. We know that stillbirth rates relating to gestational age appear as a U-shaped curve in almost every study. That is, there are higher rates of stillbirth in early pregnancy, because being born preterm is riskier, and then the stillbirth rates go down between 37 and 38 weeks of pregnancy. When the graph reaches 40 weeks, the stillbirth rates start to go up again a bit, although they remain low overall.

In 2019, a large meta-analysis on the risk of stillbirth and neonatal death was published (Muglu 2019). It included data from 13 studies and more than 15 million pregnancies. This amount of data is a significant advantage when we look at this sort of question, but there were some disadvantages too. The researchers decided to include some older studies. Several include births from the 1980s, which is forty years ago, and one went as far back as 1967. Older studies tend to have higher rates of stillbirth than more recent studies, such as Weiss *et al* (2014) and practice has changed in the past few decades. For example, better ways of monitoring babies in the womb mean that the risks are lower in populations of women giving birth now than in those who gave birth twenty years ago. And women and families need to know what the risks are now, not what they were for their mothers or grandmothers. Nonetheless, these are the most recent figures.

For all pregnancies, including those considered 'high risk', which includes multiple births (twins or more), women with medical conditions and babies with congenital abnormalities:

At 38 weeks, the risk of stillbirth was 0.16/1000, so 1 in 6250.
At 39 weeks, the risk of stillbirth was 0.42/1000, so 1 in 2380.
At 40 weeks, the risk of stillbirth was 0.69/1000, so 1 in 1450.
At 41 weeks, the risk of stillbirth was 1.66/1000, so 1 in 602.
At 42 weeks, the risk of stillbirth was 3.18/1000, so 1 in 315.
(Data from Muglu *et al* 2019).

For 'low risk' pregnancies, so a pregnancy where there is just one baby who has no congenital abnormalities and where the woman has no medical conditions:

At 38 weeks, the risk of stillbirth was 0.12/1000, so 1 in 8333.
At 39 weeks, the risk of stillbirth was 0.14/1000, so 1 in 7142.
At 40 weeks, the risk of stillbirth was 0.33/1000, so 1 in 3030.
At 41 weeks, the risk of stillbirth was 0.80/1000, so 1 in 1250.
At 42 weeks, the risk of stillbirth was 0.88/1000, so 1 in 1136.
(Data from Muglu *et al* 2019).

As you can see, the picture looks rather different if a woman/pregnancy is deemed to be 'low risk'. But I will also again remind anyone who has been labelled as 'at high risk' that maternity care has improved since researchers gathered some of the data on which these figures are based. Some babies with congenital abnormalities sadly can't be saved by any intervention. Many high-income countries have implemented initiatives to reduce stillbirth, and some of the babies who were stillborn in the years in which these data were gathered would today be identified as being in need of an induction or a caesarean for specific medical reasons and not simply because a certain date had been reached.

But does induction make a difference?

The data I shared above shows how the increased chance of stillbirth in late pregnancy is less than many people think and occurs later than many people think. But there's another really critical fact. We don't have good evidence that induction makes a difference to stillbirth rates until after 42 weeks of pregnancy. Some people will argue with this, so my plan in this section is to explain the research and you can then decide for yourself.

While the people writing guidelines tend to focus on the studies which have concluded that inducing labour before 42 weeks improves stillbirth rates, there are some individual studies (for example Rydahl *et al* 2019) and reviews of the evidence (Keulen *et al* 2018) which show that inducing labour before 42 weeks makes no difference to stillbirth rates.

These differences in outcomes exist for several reasons. One is that stillbirth is rare, no matter what you do or decide at the end of pregnancy. To see whether induction or any other intervention makes a difference to stillbirth rates, you need a very large number of woman and babies in the study, and this isn't possible in many trials. But it's clear from the body of research that any difference in outcomes before 42 completed weeks of pregnancy is marginal. In other words, if induction is beneficial, it's only slightly beneficial. That's why different studies have different results.

The fact that many of the individual studies don't show a difference between induction and expectant management before 42 completed weeks of pregnancy means that researchers add the findings of the trials together to try and get a better sense of what is happening. We call this a meta-analysis. Some meta-analyses show a small reduction in stillbirth for women whose labours are induced between 41 and 42 weeks of pregnancy (Middleton *et al* 2020). Others have found that there is no difference (Wennerholm *et al* 2009) or that the difference is marginal and the evidence about timing is weak (Coates *et al* 2020b).

Although some of the studies were of poor quality and potentially biased, most guidelines state that offering women induction before 42 weeks confers a small but statistically significant reduction in stillbirth (Wickham 2018a). That's why, for a number of years, induction has been offered in the UK and some other countries between 41 and 42 weeks of pregnancy. Not everyone wants it, but it's there as an option.

These long-standing timeframes are being challenged and changed, despite the fact that the evidence is debatable. The most recent Cochrane review and meta-analysis on this topic found, *"...a clear reduction in perinatal death with a policy of labour induction at or beyond 37 weeks compared with expectant management, though absolute rates are small (0.4 versus 3 deaths per 1000)."* (Middleton *et al* 2020).

This conclusion highlights a small but concerning change. The wording of the review has changed from discussing induction at or beyond 41 weeks to induction after 37 weeks. This illustrates the increasing move towards earlier induction, but it's not at all helpful to woman and families. Most of the data that we have relate to induction between 41 and 42 weeks and, as I've just explained, any reduction in stillbirth is small and debatable. Midwives report that, while many (though not all) women are open to induction when they near 42 weeks, most don't want induction before this point.

The authors of the latest Cochrane review (Middleton *et al* 2020) acknowledge that the absolute risk is still small and call for more research looking at how induction may affect the later neurodevelopment of children. As the Middleton *et al* (2020) review was published before Dahlen *et al*'s (2021) research on longer-term outcomes, we can hope this will be included in the next Cochrane review update.

I want to explain in a bit more depth why these differences in the conclusions exist. One reason is that the reviewers who carried out the analyses have included different studies in their meta-analysis. Why would they do that? Well, I've noted that some of the studies were conducted at a time when practice was different. Some reviewers think it's better to leave those out, and focus on recent research, carried out in settings similar to those encountered by women today. Others include the older studies as well as recent ones. Researchers also use different definitions of 'low risk,' and the protocols (which are the procedures and practices used in research projects, which tell clinicians things such as when and how to monitor the wellbeing of babies) vary between studies. Some recent reviewers have taken account of these factors and have been more selective about the studies they include. But other reviewers have included all of the studies. There's not a right or wrong way to decide such things, either. These are human decisions, and people's viewpoints vary.

As one example, Keulen *et al* (2018) addressed the question of using different time frames for induction. They set out to see whether there was a difference between elective induction of labour and expectant management if we just look at studies within the 41–42 weeks' timeframe. Their conclusion was different from that of the Middleton *et al* (2020) review. Keulen *et al* (2018) concluded that, *"Evidence is lacking for the recommendation to induce labour at 41 weeks instead of 42 weeks for the improvement of perinatal outcome."*

Rydahl *et al* (2019) also set out to look more thoughtfully at which studies should be included in a meta-analysis. They focused on recent studies (within the past 20 years) which compared healthy (or low risk) women having induction at 41 and 42 weeks. Again, they found no difference in perinatal mortality, morbidity and caesarean section rates.

"Induction prior to post-term was associated with few beneficial outcomes and several adverse outcomes. This draws attention to possible iatrogenic effects affecting large numbers of low-risk women in contemporary maternity care. According to the World Health Organization, expected benefits from a medical intervention must outweigh potential harms. Hence, our results do not support the widespread use of routine induction prior to post-term (41+0–6 gestational weeks)." (Rydahl *et al* 2019: 170).

Another reason why reviews and summaries are helpful is because individual studies can sometimes be misleading, or flawed. This doesn't stop them from making headlines, however. A good example of this is the SWEPIS study. This was a Swedish trial on comparing induction of labour at 41 weeks with expectant management. The study was stopped before it was finished because of a significantly higher rate of perinatal mortality in the babies born to the women having expectant management (Wennerholm *et al* 2019). While some proponents of induction were quick to cite this as evidence of the risks of late pregnancy, a number of long-time experts on induction trials, research design and statistics pointed out that this conclusion could not be drawn. Some wrote that the decision to stop the trial was based on flawed logic (Timpka & Larsson 2019) and one long-time induction researcher explained that the *"...trial suffer*[s] *from serious errors owing to conduct, analysis and reporting."* (Olsen 2019).

It's relatively easy these days to find a study to support anything you want to claim is evidence-based. But that's not what the original proponents of evidence-based medicine were aiming for. The real understanding comes from reviewing the wider body of evidence, considering the pros and cons of the study designs and understanding that there's always a bigger picture. As I keep saying, it's complicated. But it's worth taking time to understand in depth.

What's not compared, and who's not included?

Not everyone is represented in induction research. Most studies compare expectant management with induction of labour at a certain point in pregnancy. Most studies are also carried out in hospitals, where practice is often medically focused. But not everyone will have this type of care.

For example, some women have independent midwives or private obstetricians. Some freebirth, and choose to have no professional caregiver. There are those who opt for hospital-based care but choose not to have expectant management, for instance by not turning up for appointments because they don't want to be monitored in this way. Some women avoid the maternity services or turn up at the last minute, perhaps because they are refugees and are afraid of reprisal. They might not speak the language of the country they are in, or know that care is available. There are women who have hospital care but who decline routine induction. Some of those women might make a care plan with their own midwife or with a consultant midwife, based on a discussion of their individual situation and options. This list is not exhaustive.

So the research findings discussed in this chapter don't necessarily apply to those seeking different kinds of care, or those who don't access maternity care at all. They may not even be applicable to some of those who do seek 'standard' care. Another group of women who aren't included in induction research are the women who were invited to participate in the studies, but who decided not to. This is well explained by Kenyon *et al* (2019). They point out that, as well as being insufficiently powered – i.e. there weren't enough women and babies to assess perinatal mortality – and not looking at long-term outcomes, trials may struggle to recruit women, and this may be significant.

"…discussion was provoked by the large numbers of eligible women who declined to participate in both trials, and the same occurred in the [INDEX] trial by Keulen and colleagues: more than 6000 women had to be approached to achieve the recruitment target of 1800. This might indicate that those who did participate were different from the general population, and the authors highlight that this trial included mainly white women younger than 35 years." (Kenyon *et al* 2019).

The fact that as many as three quarters of the women who are invited to participate in induction trials decline to do so is important. It implies that many women have a preference for either spontaneous or induced labour (Kenyon *et al* 2019). It means that induction trials contain a self-selected sample, and it's another reason why we can't put much store in claims that women in such studies were satisfied with induction. Women don't agree to take part in such studies if they want to avoid induction. Some enter the study because it gives them a chance of earlier induction that they wouldn't otherwise get. Nothing wrong with that if that's what you prefer, but we need to avoid falling into the trap of thinking that the views of those in induction studies are representative of everyone.

One reason to be aware of this is that some obstetricians claim that the idea that women don't like induction, *"...is not borne out by the evidence"* (Lightly & Weeks 2020). The obstetricians who made this statement in an opinion piece gave one reference to a study whose authors wrote a response stating that Lightly & Weeks' (2020) had made *"...inaccurate representations"* about their review (Coates *et al* 2019). As I showed in chapter three, the evidence on what women think, feel and want is complex, and we need to remember that the trials don't represent the experience of all women. In fact, many groups, including Black, Brown, Asian and mixed race women, aren't well represented in induction research at all.

But what about the ARRIVE trial?

In recent years, I have been asked one induction-related question more than any other. It goes like this:

"I saw the consultant, said I didn't want induction. He quoted the ARRIVE trial at me and told me that induction was better because it leads to fewer caesareans. That doesn't make sense to me, because about three quarters of the women I know who had an induction ended up with a caesarean. What's going on?" (Charlie).

The ARRIVE trial (Grobman *et al* 2018) was a study carried out in the USA. The researchers looked at whether inducing labour in healthy women at 39 weeks of pregnancy led to a lower caesarean rate compared to awaiting spontaneous labour. The results suggested that induction reduced the chance of caesarean and this finding is often quoted in support of earlier induction. However, a great many people and papers have questioned the validity of the findings of the ARRIVE trial, which contains many sources of possible bias (Dahlen personal correspondence 2018, Davies-Tuck *et al* 2018, Goer 2018, Wickham 2018a, King *et al* 2019, Scialli 2019a,

2019b). Some point to the large body of research showing that induction increases the chance of caesarean (Butler *et al* 1993, Johantgen *et al* 2012, Sandall *et al* 2016, Saccone *et al* 2019, Souter *et al* 2019b, Reed 2019a, Declerq *et al* 2020). Others have criticised colleagues for over-simplifying and over-stating the findings of this trial (Glantz 2019). I don't think the ARRIVE trial is very useful as a means of informing decisions about induction. But sometimes we can learn more from the less valid studies than the robust ones. The detail and story of the ARRIVE trial helps show how current recommendations are based as much on myth as on robust evidence.

A key thing to know is that the ARRIVE trial does not show that induction improves outcomes for babies. It did set out to look at that but, as with many induction studies, there was no difference in outcomes between the two groups. So induction at 39 weeks confers no short-term benefit to babies.

One of the secondary outcomes that the ARRIVE trial researchers looked at was whether induction makes caesarean more or less likely. And their results do seem to show that induction at 39 weeks of pregnancy is associated with a lower caesarean rate than expectant management. In the induction group, 18.6% of women had a caesarean, compared to 22.2% in the expectant management group.

That's not much of a difference, although it's possible to spin the results of any study. Obstetrician J Christopher Glantz (2019) wrote about this. He pointed out that the ARRIVE trial is just one study, yet some doctors were (and still are) overstating the results, without explaining the flaws in the research.

"What is inappropriate is taking one study at face value and expressing likelihoods in a manner that inflates their benefit. Lowering the ceserean delivery rate by 16% sounds impressive; a 3.6 percentage point decrease - or that 28 inductions would be required to prevent one caesarean delivery – sounds much less so." (Glantz 2019: 179).

There are also issues with the design of the ARRIVE trial. Many of the women who were asked to participate declined to do so, as discussed above. So the trial included only one rather narrow group. There also wasn't much difference in the average gestational age at birth between the two groups. Women in the induction group gave birth on average at 39 weeks and three days. Women in the expectant management group gave birth on average at 40 weeks, which is only four days different. That may partly be because 280 of the 3044 women in the expectant management group actually had their labour induced early, although the study protocol was not followed for 366 of the 3062 women in the early induction group either. It's not clear exactly what happened there, and whether some of the women waited for spontaneous labour.

Expert maternity researcher Henci Goer describes how a higher proportion of the women developed hypertension or pre-eclampsia over the period of the study than we would expect from looking at the proportion of women who normally develop these conditions. She explained that it's unclear whether the ARRIVE trial was genuinely studying women with a low risk pregnancy or whether these diagnoses were given to justify induction of labour in some of the women in the control group (Goer 2018). *"In short, control-group women weren't playing on a level playing field, and a case can be made that investigators were interpreting the data to fit their pre-conceived notions."* (Goer 2018).

A letter from some of those involved in the ARRIVE trial states that they, *"…feel that performing 28 inductions to prevent one caesarean delivery is better than anything we currently have to prevent cesarean deliveries."* (Marrs *et al* 2019). But a lot of research shows that continuity of midwifery care leads to equally good or better survival rates for babies while increasing the likelihood of physiological birth and reducing caesareans; both in the USA where the ARRIVE trial was carried out, and around the world (Butler *et al* 1993, Johantgen *et al* 2012, Sandall *et al* 2016, Souter *et al* 2019b, Reed 2019a, Declerq *et al* 2020). And, as one midwife said:

"It's a little staggering that, when they realise that there isn't any benefit in terms of perinatal mortality, and they can't find the

one thing they were looking for, they instead look for and report another. So now we have induction being sold as a means to normal birth, which is sort of hilarious – because there's nothing normal about induced labour – and sort of tragic, because you just know what's going to happen to all these poor women." (Jenn).

The deeper one dug, the more things came to light. Hannah Dahlen (personal correspondence 2019) pointed out that the caesarean section rate was very high in both groups, especially given that these women were deemed to have a low risk pregnancy. In fact, the women's care was generally very medicalised, and 94% were cared for by private obstetricians, which means that the findings aren't applicable to settings where this isn't the case (Davies-Tuck *et al* 2018, Wickham 2018a, Reed 2019a, Souter *et al* 2019a).

Does induction decrease the chance of caesarean?

Contrary to the ARRIVE trial and one or two other studies, many studies show the opposite finding about caesarean sections. There is abundant evidence from research and real-world data that induction does not decrease the caesarean section rate, but actually increases it (Zhao *et al* 2017, Rydahl *et al* 2019, Gunnarsdóttir *et al* 2021, Levine *et al* 2021, Espada-Trespalacios *et al* 2021). This is especially the case for women who are labouring for the first time (Davey & King 2016, Kjerulff *et al* 2017). Other studies such as the review that I cited above find, *"…no significant difference in the Caesarean section rate 93/629 (induction) versus 106/629 (expectant management)."* (Keulan *et al* 2018). It's important to understand why different studies come up with different findings about induction and caesarean rates, and why caesarean section rates aren't a very reliable outcome measure.

The question of whether induction of labour increases or decreases the caesarean rate in a research study depends on what you're measuring, who you're including, and what you're comparing (Wickham 2018a, Bhide 2021). For instance, as Rachel Reed (2019a) highlighted, *"…most research comparing induction with spontaneous labour combines populations of 'experienced' labourers with first timers."* This 'comparing apples with oranges' approach is just one reason why the findings of different trials, studies, reviews and commentaries vary.

Another issue is that, if you compare induction with spontaneous labour, then women who have inductions definitely have a much higher chance of ending up with a caesarean. Women like Charlie, who I quoted above, see every day that those whose labours are induced in systems of modern maternity care are more likely to end in a caesarean than those who wait. But if you compare induction with the obstetrically defined approach to 'expectant management,' then planned induction does seem to carry a lower chance of caesarean section in some studies (Grobman *et al* 2018, Bhide 2021, Zenzmaier *et al* 2021). But what does expectant management mean in this context, and why might this be happening? And how can a particular approach to 'expectant management' make planned induction less likely to lead to a caesarean in studies when those working in maternity hospitals witness the cascade of intervention that tends to follow induced labour lead to caesareans every single day?

To answer that question, we need to understand how humans affect research.

How human decisions affect research findings

If you want to measure or compare two or more things in a research study – like drugs or approaches to the end of pregnancy – then you need to define what you're going to use as outcome measures. In other words, what you'll measure in order to know whether there's a difference between the groups you're researching.

Some outcome measures are easy to agree on. In some studies, we measure things like whether somebody is alive or not at a certain point. There is a tiny grey area in which it's hard to agree. Someone can be alive on a life support machine who wouldn't be alive without it. But mostly the answer is clear. It's the same with other kinds of measurements. Did the flight land on time? Did the temperature rise above 20 degrees? As long as the definitions and instruments are standardised, these things are easy to measure and agree on. Researchers call these 'hard' outcome measures. In a nutshell, we don't have to worry so much about subjectivity, or how human emotions, experiences and differences of opinion might affect the assessment of the outcomes.

But in maternity research, we use a lot of outcome measures that are subjective, or dependent on individual opinion. And 'is a caesarean necessary at this point in time?' is a good example of this. Professional opinions differ.

"…we need to be aware that it is humans who make the decision to do a caesarean, or the decision to induce labour in a woman who is in the control group. So this trial isn't measuring the natural outcome of a labour; it may say more about medical decision making and the level of intervention preferred by those who were involved in the study." (Wickham 2018a: 54)

Some practitioners will have a much higher or lower tolerance for certain situations, and this depends on many individual factors. Main *et al* (2020) showed that how doctors practice individually and how a hospital usually does things influence the experiences of healthy women having their first baby. A formal survey of obstetricians' attitudes to the idea of earlier induction showed wide variation (Davis *et al* 2021), as do the quotes in this book from doctors and midwives. Just as many are speaking out against routine induction as for it.

An interesting issue was raised by Scialli (2019a), who describes himself as an obstetrician of a certain vintage. He sees how practice has changed in recent years, and that his more impatient colleagues may now be faster to recommend induction and caesarean. He describes how those of his era might have used patience and skill to restore balance so women could give birth themselves and in their own time:

"The studies in this area are limited by the expectant management group being managed by modern obstetricians, whose

inclination for intervention may be higher than is optimal. Larger babies mean longer labors, which may tax the patience of the modern obstetricians, and preeclampsia is alarming to some practitioners who may not be willing to stabilize the patient and wait for the uterus to respond to oxytocin. As gestation advances, there may be less amniotic fluid with consequent benign variable decelerations that are over-interpreted as fetal hypoxemia.

The answer might come from a careful review of the cesarean deliveries in these studies to determine whether they represent a disadvantage of expectant management or a consequence of modern obstetrics training. Obstetricians of my vintage were trained when the cesarean delivery rate was considered high at 15% and when we didn't have so many categories of fetal tracings. Even in the modern era, the midwives at my institution have a cesarean delivery rate of 3–5%, caring for exactly the kind of patient in the ARRIVE trial. The current high induction and cesarean rates in modern obstetrics have not given us better babies, and we would do well to be concerned about effects on maternal morbidity and mortality rates." (Scialli 2019a: 79).

In summary, the offer of a caesarean is a clinical decision based on the obstetrician's beliefs and biases as well as evidence and experience. So studies that use caesarean rates as an outcome measure are measuring the practitioner's beliefs and fears rather than how many women might have given birth to a healthy baby spontaneously if they had had more time. Many practitioners are worried about post-term pregnancy, despite the evidence. They've been taught to be worried, and this can lead them to recommend caesarean earlier in a woman in spontaneous labour at 41 weeks than someone in induced labour at 39 weeks. They are more anxious about 'post-dates' pregnancy and feel more in control when someone's labour is being medically managed, which may mean they have a lower threshold for intervention.

Some people do acknowledge that the caesarean risk changes depending on how we define expectant management (Bhide 2021). But it is frustratingly difficult to get others to understand that their own bias and fear combined with how the research on induction is designed and where birth usually takes place may have a bigger impact on induction and caesarean rates than factors to do with the woman and baby.

It's rather shocking to realise just how much of the current conversation and practices are based on belief rather than evidence. When it comes to some of what is being shared about the pros and cons of induction in late pregnancy, what we're seeing isn't evidence-based decision making. It's decision-based evidence making. This makes it all the more important that women and families can explore the evidence and the issues for themselves, so that they can make the decisions that are right for them.

Overall, the evidence on induction for post-term pregnancy shows that, while induction may be associated with a small reduction in the risk of stillbirth in very late pregnancy, there's no benefit in relation to stillbirth rates until pregnancy nears 42 weeks. The fact that induction carries risks and disadvantages means that, no matter when induction is offered, this decision needs to be carefully considered as part of a bigger picture. As Seijmonsbergen-Schermers *et al* (2019) note, *"...all induced women will be exposed to potential disadvantages ... Offering induction to all women at term ignores the principles of the Hippocratic oath, 'first, do no harm."*

6. Does my baby look big in thi

"If I could change one thing about my pregnancy, it would be to not have the scan where they estimated the baby's size and said he was going to be big. They immediately wanted to induce me and even though I said no at first, they broke me down with the pressure. And the induction itself wasn't as bad as it is for some women, I know, but when he was born he was just over seven pounds, so hardly big. And I'll always wonder, did you need a bit more time in there, mate? What are we doing by making all these babies come before they're ready?" (Xanthe).

"I was told that Xavian would be around the 7lb mark. He was 8lb 12. Kairo was then 'feared' to be over 8lbs. He was born 5lbs 5. They then told me Zaria was also measuring small the whole pregnancy and would likely be around the same birth weight as Kairo. She was born 8lbs 2." (Leah).

Xanthe, Leah and thousands of women like them are telling a story of our time. Go to any parent and baby group in a country where scans are used routinely, and you'll hear similar tales. There is increasing emphasis on measuring babies in the womb by ultrasound. If a baby is estimated to be large for its age, additional screening may be recommended, and induction may be offered. The medical term for a large baby is macrosomia and, because this now affects so many families, that's what I'm going to discuss in this chapter.

Induction is offered in this situation in the hope of preventing an occasional but sometimes serious situation called shoulder dystocia, which I'll explain below. But there isn't good evidence that induction helps prevent shoulder dystocia or the problems it can sometimes lead to. We do know that these offers of induction for 'suspected large baby' or for a baby considered to be 'large for dates' or 'large for gestational age' (LGA) are creating a huge amount of anxiety and stress for women and families, though. Induction for any reason carries all the potential risks and downsides that I've discussed in previous chapters, so the benefits and risks need to be carefully weighed up in each individual situation. But one of the most significant issues when it comes to suspected big babies, as you'll already know from Xanthe and Leah, is that ultrasounds are often wrong.

What's the problem?

Shoulder dystocia is one of those occasional but rarely serious situations. It's the term we use for when a baby's shoulder gets stuck during birth and they need extra help to be born. Shoulder dystocia happens in about one in 200 births, and the UK's Health and Safety Investigation Branch (HSIB) estimate that 3,770 to 4,550 cases of shoulder dystocia occur in England each year. That might sound like a lot, but midwives and doctors are well-trained in dealing with shoulder dystocia. There are special movements and manoeuvres that help the baby out, and the majority of cases of shoulder dystocia will resolve with one simple manoeuvre and don't result in any injury or problem (HSIB 2020). A small number of babies experience a birth injury after shoulder dystocia. In the worst-case scenario, shoulder dystocia can lead to brain damage or very rarely death, but these are very rare consequences.

The theory behind the suggested intervention is that a larger baby is more likely to get stuck at birth. So if we offer inductions for 'large for dates' babies, maybe we can prevent most cases of shoulder dystocia from happening in the first place. A statistic of concern to those organising maternity care is that, when these very occasional and serious consequences do occur as a result of shoulder dystocia, they are a leading cause of doctors and hospitals getting sued (RCOG 2012a). Many women and families report being coerced by fearful professionals, so I think it's important to mention this legal aspect. Offering induction for suspected large babies may be more about hospitals' fear of litigation than there being evidence that intervention helps prevent shoulder dystocia.

This is another example of something which affects only a few women and babies, but where we're offering intervention to lots of people 'just in case'. Whether or not to have an induction for a suspected big baby is a personal decision. In order to make the decision, people need clear information about the chance of something happening, the effectiveness of the intervention at preventing it and, of course, the downsides of induction, which I've discussed elsewhere in this book. Let's have a look at the evidence.

Defining big babies

The first issue is that the thing we're screening for – large babies – is actually quite common. The definition of a large baby varies a bit. Many organisations define a large baby as one who weighs more than 4kg at birth, which is 8lb 13oz. But, as Rachel Reed (2019b) writes:

"Big babies are normal in well resourced countries. Over 10% of babies born in the UK and Australia weigh 4kg (8lb 13oz) or more. Healthy well nourished women grow healthy well nourished babies. Genetic factors also influence the size of babies (big babies run in families); and each baby a woman has usually weighs more than the last. Babies also continue to grow at the end of pregnancy (because placentas continue to nourish them rather than switch off) – so a baby will be bigger at 42 weeks than they were at 40 weeks."

Like with length of pregnancy, we know that big babies are associated with a few other factors. These factors include maternal age and size, weight gain in pregnancy and maternal diabetes (Cameron *et al* 2014, Gaudet *et al* 2014, Fang *et al* 2019, Rui-Xhe *et al* 2019). But not every woman who has diabetes or any other factor will have a large baby.

I mentioned above that suspected large babies are sometimes described as 'large for gestational age,' or LGA. A baby is generally described as being LGA if it weighs more than 90% of babies who are of the same gestational age (Rouse *et al* 1996). We also call this being 'above the 90th centile', and this phrase is commonly heard where growth charts are used.

Centiles, averages and normality

It's important to note though, that being above the 90th centile or being labelled as such doesn't necessarily mean you have a problem. My husband's height is above the 90th centile, and this isn't a hindrance unless you count the number of times he bangs his head in low-beamed cottages. In many situations, being an outlier can actually be an advantage. He is beloved by little old ladies in supermarkets, because he will happily reach things on high shelves for them. In another example, most of the New Zealand All Blacks rugby players have a BMI (or body mass index, supposedly a measure of how overweight you are) which puts them in the 'obese' category. Yet they are world class athletes.

Western medicine is based on ideas about measuring aspects of people and putting us into categories which then determine whether we are perceived to be 'at risk.' But there's often no correlation between falling into (or outside of) a particular category and having a problem or condition. This tendency to put people into categories based on just one aspect of their health or size is another consequence of the reductionist approach that I described in chapter two. We need to take a much broader approach to assessing and supporting health and wellbeing, and not simply focus on one factor, such as size. Especially in situations where size is estimated and our estimations are often wrong, or have a margin of error.

Many midwives and birth workers see this happening every day, and they often describe feeling frustrated at the message, both direct and indirect, that women and families are being given.

"I think the biggest thing that I'm trying to get my head around is induction for predicted LGA babies. I don't think women are getting balanced information about induction for LGA. So many women I look after are otherwise low risk and are having inductions for babies who end up being average size." (Fiona, midwife).

"The other part that often is forgotten in the discussions with women is that it may be normal for them to produce a big baby and

not have any problems birthing said baby. It's like everyone forgets that GROW charts are all about normal distribution and that there are always going to be babies who weigh more or less than considered normal!" (Terri, midwife).

The assumptions and the evidence

A number of assumptions are linked in an attempt to justify induction for suspected large babies just as assumptions about post-term pregnancy are linked to justify induction in that situation, as I described in chapters four and five. In the case of suspected big babies, the first assumption is the idea that there is a link between the size of a baby and their chance of getting shoulder dystocia. If this were the case, it might help us to successfully predict when shoulder dystocia might happen, although we would then still have to find an effective means of preventing it. But in reality there isn't a strong enough link between baby size and the chances of shoulder dystocia, which means we can't use estimated fetal size as a means of knowing which babies might experience this particular complication.

It is true that, on average, a large baby is more likely to experience shoulder dystocia than a small baby. But we have long known that most large babies are born without experiencing this (Gross *et al* 1987, RCOG 2012a). Another key and long understood fact is that many cases of shoulder dystocia occur in babies who are of average size or who are even smaller than average (Baskett & Allen 1995, RCOG 2012a, Nath *et al* 2015). A study by Beta *et al* (2019) showed that only 6% of the babies who weighed more than 4kg experienced shoulder dystocia. This means that 94% of babies weighing more than 4kg didn't experience this. So one in 17 of the babies who weigh more than 4kg at birth experience shoulder dystocia, and the other 16 are fine. This is babies who are actually over 4kg, by the way, not those who are predicted as being over 4kg. I will discuss the inaccuracy of ultrasound weight estimation in the next section.

We do know that rates of shoulder dystocia are higher in women who have poorly controlled diabetes (Rouse *et al* 1996, Reed 2019b). This is an example of the kind of situation where induction might be beneficial to some women and babies, although another option is to focus on getting the diabetes under control during pregnancy. But assessment and decision making still needs to be individual, as many babies in this situation will be fine too. Remember also that most babies who experience shoulder dystocia won't suffer any long-term consequences from this and that, as we saw from previous chapters, induction carries downsides as well as benefits. As does the screening itself, but I'll come back to that later.

In summary, no study has been able to accurately predict which babies will experience shoulder dystocia (Leung *et al* 2011, RCOG 2012a, Boulvain *et al* 2016) and no study has been able to predict which of the babies who experience shoulder dystocia will be negatively affected as a result of this (RCOG 2012a, Boulvain *et al* 2016).

Estimating the baby's weight

But there's another big and problematic assumption, and it's to do with the accuracy of trying to predict the size of a baby in pregnancy. Measuring babies in a woman's womb with our hands or with a tape measure is accurate only half the time (Chauhan *et al* 2005). As with due dates, ultrasound isn't very accurate at predicting a baby's size either. Most studies and reviews show that there is a margin of error of 15% either way (Rossi *et al* 2013, Boulvain *et al* 2016, Milner & Arezina 2018).

Anecdotally, some midwives, doctors and sonographers think that the margin of error is even wider than this in real life. That's because some of the studies are done under 'ideal' conditions and people may take more care than usual because they know their work is being measured. It's also sometimes the case that the measurements are taken in centres of excellence. That's not to disrespect professionals or suggest they aren't doing their best every day. But it's easy to fall into patterns or to miss things when you're doing the same thing repeatedly, or when people are interrupting and talking to you and there's more noise than is experienced when reading an ultrasound scan in a quiet room during a research study.

So for a baby estimated to weigh 4kg (the cut-off point usually used to define suspected macrosomia), a 15% margin either side means the range of the estimate is from 3400g (7lbs 5oz) to 4600g (10lbs 4oz). That's quite a range. And it's still only an estimate, not a guarantee. A few babies will weigh more or less than a weight that falls within the 15% margin.

Curiously, professionals seem more likely to overestimate than underestimate. The researchers in the 'Listening to Mothers' survey that I shared in chapter three looked at this issue as well. They found that one in three women were told their baby was 'too big' based on ultrasound, and yet the actual average birth weight of the babies who were suspected of being big was 7lb 13oz or 3590g (Cheng *et al* 2015). Midwives also describe seeing many babies who weigh less than the ultrasound-estimated birth weight.

"I notice the weight guess on the scan is often wrong. Time and again we see induction being booked for large or small babies and the actual weight is way off. I think it SEEMS really accurate partly because it comes from the high-tech scan department on a fancy graph print out and also because they print it down to the last gram. So you would have estimated fetal weight of for example 3462g. The way it is put so precisely makes it seem more accurate in a way than for instance a measure of 3.2 to 3.6 kg." (Andie, midwife).

As Rachel Reed (2019b) says, *"The only way to accurately assess the weight of a baby is to weigh them after birth."*

Is induction for suspected big babies beneficial?

We know that the screening methods that we're using to estimating a baby's weight by ultrasound aren't effective at identifying (a) enough of the babies who are LGA, and (b) only the babies who are LGA. The idea that we can identify suspected large babies by ultrasound and then prevent shoulder dystocia by offering early induction to babies suspected to be larger than average isn't evidence-based.

Another consideration is whether there is evidence that, if we offer early induction, it improves outcomes. The simple answer to this question is no. We don't have much evidence to help us answer this question. The Cochrane review on macrosomia (Boulvain *et al* 2016) showed that only 1100 women have ever been involved in trials. This isn't a large number given that shoulder dystocia is relatively rare and serious outcomes from shoulder dystocia are even rarer. When adverse outcomes are rare, we need larger trials to be able to see if screening or intervention makes a difference. Their meta-analysis found that induction in mothers with suspected large for gestational age babies reduced the number of babies who had shoulder dystocia from 6.8% with expectant management to 4.1% in the induction group. But there were no differences in the kind of birth injury that researchers were looking at.

"No clear differences between groups were reported for damage to the network of nerves that send signals from the spine to the shoulder, arm and hand (brachial plexus injury) of the baby (low-quality evidence due to very few events occurring) or signs of not enough oxygen during birth. A policy of labour induction reduced the average birthweight of babies by 178 g. The trials did not show any differences in the number of women who had caesarean sections or instrumental births. There is limited evidence that more women in the induction of labour group had severe damage to the perineum. We conclude that there appear to be benefits, but there may also be some disadvantages of induction of labour shortly before term." (Boulvain *et al* 2016).

In the analysis the authors found another disadvantage to being born too early; the babies whose mothers' labours were induced had a greater chance of being jaundiced. I'd also like to point out the line in there about the difference in average birthweight between the two groups. As I am fond of saying, 178g is the weight of the average hamster, or a medium sized pear (Wickham 2018a). Not a big difference at all.

Boulvain *et al* (2016) also noted that, *"…antenatal estimates of fetal weight are often inaccurate so many women may be worried unnecessarily, and many inductions may not be needed."*

In another review of the evidence, Coates *et al* (2020b) looked at more than 300 research papers which had assessed common indications for induction of labour. In other words, they carried out an assessment of research relating to the many different reasons for which induction is offered. They also found no evidence that induction was beneficial for suspected macrosomia.

The lack of evidence of benefit, and the lack of much evidence on this at all means that researchers, including Boulvain *et al* (2016), have been calling for a randomised controlled trial on this topic. A 'Big Baby Trial' is currently underway. The researchers running it also acknowledge that, at present, there is no evidence to support induction for big babies in their explanation of how the trial will work:

"Currently it is not clear whether it is better for women with big babies to have their labour induced or to wait for labour to begin naturally. To answer this question a clinical trial is needed. We propose to study 4,000 pregnant women whose ultrasound scans suggests [sic] *that their babies are bigger than expected. With the woman's consent, she will be allocated at random to either have an induction of labour at 38 weeks or to wait until labour starts naturally. We will compare outcomes between the two groups to look at whether, as a result of induction of labour at about 38 weeks, there were fewer complications such as shoulder dystocia. There will also be a parallel Cohort Study of women who decline to be randomised (for example if the woman requests a Caesarean section) but would consent for us to study their delivery information."* (Warwick Clinical Trials Unit 2021).

Anecdotally, midwives and doctors in the hospitals where the trial is taking place are reporting that, just as with some of the induction trials that I discussed in chapter five, many women are declining to enter the trial. On the whole, this is not because they want a caesarean. It's because they do not want the onset of their labour to be decided randomly, or they don't want to take the chance of having to have induction at 38 weeks. The results of this trial will be interesting, not just in what they can tell us about whether there is a difference between induction and expectant management when babies are thought to be large. It will also be interesting to see whether the Big Baby Trial is beset by the same issues and sources of potential bias as some of the other induction trials.

Downsides of inducing for suspected big babies

The most significant downside to offering early induction to anyone whose baby is suspected to be large involves the risks of induction, which I've already discussed elsewhere. Additionally, women whose labour is induced for suspected macrosomia may be at even higher risk of being told they need a caesarean than women offered induction for other reasons. Research in Australia showed that, for a woman having her first baby, the chance of having a caesarean after induction varied according to the reason for induction (de Vries *et al* 2019). In that study, the women most likely to end up with a caesarean were those whose labours were being induced for a suspected large baby.

This might not be anything to do with the size of the baby or the ability of the woman to birth it. As I discussed in chapter five, caesarean is a clinical decision and not a natural outcome. This could be about the practitioners' fear rather than anything to do with the woman's body.

The downsides of screening

Women and families also need to know that even having a scan itself can have downsides. Once a baby has been labelled or diagnosed as big, pressure may be put on the woman to accept interventions. Even if the woman declines induction, she may be told that certain options (for instance birthing at home or in a birth centre) are no longer open to her. There is no evidence to support this recommendation and in most countries no-one can stop a woman staying at home to give birth, but it's something that I hear often.

Reed (2019b) has summarised evidence showing that the perception of a baby's size influences outcomes more than the actual size of the baby:

"… research suggests that the complications associated with big babies may be due to interventions carried out when a baby is suspected to be big. Care providers are more likely to diagnose slow progress during labour and recommend a caesarean if they suspect the baby is big (Blackwell et al 2009). Women who are told that they have a 'big baby', and are counselled about potential complications, are significantly more likely to choose a planned caesarean (Peleg et al 2015). One study compared the outcomes of a group of women with suspected big babies with a group of women who unexpectedly gave birth to a big baby (Sadeh-Mestechkin et al 2008). Women who were suspected of having a big baby were three times more likely to have an induction or caesarean, and were four times more likely to have complications such as severe perineal tearing and postpartum haemorrhage. In this study there were no differences in the incidence of shoulder dystocia between the two groups. Therefore, when a baby is suspected of being big, a woman has an increased chance of interventions during birth, and of experiencing complications caused by those interventions, even if the baby is not actually big… The research about complications relating to big babies suggests that it is the interventions carried out when a baby is assumed to be big – rather than the actual size of the baby – that mostly contributes to complications." (Reed 2019b)

This appears to confirm that even having a scan can itself lead to unwanted consequences. This is one reason why it's important to think through all the tests and interventions that are offered in pregnancy. Unwanted consequences of some screening tests, like ultrasound, are not always immediately apparent (Wickham 2018a, 2018b, 2019).

The recommendations and the reality

Some of the guidelines making recommendations as to what should be offered within systems of maternity care do acknowledge the uncertainty in this area, and the fact that there's no good evidence on which to base a recommendation for induction for a suspected big baby. Several guidelines also actively advise against using ultrasound screening to estimate a baby's size, and suggest that women shouldn't be offered induction of labour just for a suspected big baby.

For example, the NICE (2008b) antenatal care for uncomplicated pregnancies guideline (which is still the most recent guideline at the time of writing, despite its age) states that *"...ultrasound estimation of a baby's size for suspected LGA babies should not be undertaken in a low-risk population."* The RCOG (2012a) shoulder dystocia guideline determines that, *"...induction of labour does not prevent shoulder dystocia in nondiabetic mothers with a suspected LGA baby."* And the NICE (2008a) induction of labour guideline contained the recommendation that, *"...in the absence of any other indications induction of labour should not be carried out simply because a health professional suspects a baby is larger."* The later NICE (2021b) updated guidance now states that, *"...women should be provided with information about different modes of birth so they can make an informed decision, and that recruitment into relevant clinical trials should be supported."*

Offering an ultrasound in late pregnancy to estimate or assess the baby's size is also not supported by evidence. Wastlund *et al* (2019) found that, *"...universal late-pregnancy ultrasound screening for fetal macrosomia is not warranted."* This finding was echoed the following year by another research team, who showed that:

"Universal third-trimester ultrasound screening will identify more pregnancies with macrosomia. However, it will not have a clinically significant effect at predicting shoulder dystocia. There is not enough evidence on the effect of ultrasound screening on neonatal morbidity." Moraitis *et al* (2020).

In Australia, Neel *et al* (2021) demonstrated that a routine third trimester growth ultrasound in pregnant women with a BMI of 35 kg/m^2 or more does not reliably identify fetal growth abnormalities.

Despite the evidence, midwives and doctors from around the world tell me that women are often offered an ultrasound in late pregnancy to see if their baby is larger than average. They also report that, while efforts are being made in some areas to avoid recommending induction based on estimated size alone, fearful care providers will simply find another reason to recommend induction. Women will be told that their blood pressure is a bit high, or that the combination of their age and a possible large baby and the fact that they are themselves a bit larger than average means that, *"…it's best to be safe rather than sorry."* This is coercive, and the fear isn't based on evidence. The evidence doesn't show that induction reduces the chance of the complications that may stem from shoulder dystocia. Unnecessary intervention (or doing 'too much too soon') often causes more problems than it solves.

There's also a big flaw in the logic which I think it's worth knowing about. Near the beginning of this chapter, I quoted Rachel Reed, who discussed how placentas continue to nourish the baby towards the end of pregnancy. This highlights a fallacy in the obstetric arguments about induction for different reasons. When it comes to offering induction towards the end of pregnancy, women are often told that their placenta may fail to nourish their baby. But women (and sometimes the same women) are also being told that their baby may get too big if they wait. It's clear that these things can't both be true.

The roads less travelled

There is one more issue that I want to address before I end this chapter. If we go back to the root problem that we're trying to solve, which is preventing shoulder dystocia, it's important to understand that there are a number of ways that we may be able to prevent this which do not involve induction of labour or other invasive procedures.

For example, it may make a difference if women weren't on a bed in labour and/or 'tied' by drips and monitors. If women were encouraged and supported to move about, to get into the positions they instinctively wanted to, to use water, to push when they wanted to do so and not when someone else directed them to, this might make a positive difference. That's certainly the experience of many midwives. We see that, when we can enable women to follow their instincts, to give birth in a way that is orchestrated by their own hormones and not managed by someone else, this can be beneficial. Birthing in an upright position or on all fours often means that shoulder dystocia is prevented, as the woman's pelvis is free to move, unlike when she is sitting or lying on her back on a bed. Why aren't we researching these things more, especially when they don't have the same kind of associated downsides that pharmaceutical and technological options carry?

I'm not arguing that a change of position or a birth pool is always the answer. Shoulder dystocia can happen even when everything goes amazingly well, and I noted above that it can also happen when the baby is smaller than average. I want to mention again that there are other important factors relating to larger babies, for instance poorly controlled diabetes, which is another reason to make recommendations and decisions on an individual basis, while taking account of the whole picture. But we should be looking more widely at this problem rather than focusing in on interventions that involve large amounts of pharmaceutical drugs and a high chance of surgical intervention and that carry risks and downsides for women and babies without evidence of benefit.

As I've shown in this chapter, there are serious flaws in the idea of offering induction for a suspected big baby. It isn't supported by the evidence. We can't accurately predict the weight of a baby. Even if we could, weight isn't directly correlated with the chance of shoulder dystocia, and most babies who experience shoulder dystocia are fine. Most babies who are larger than average will be born easily, especially if their mothers are able to move about as they want to and have the kind of care which helps optimise the physiology of labour.

There's just no evidence that screening for macrosomia, telling women that their baby is thought to be larger than average (while omitting to mention that there is a margin of error in the estimation) and offering induction when a baby is suspected to be larger than average is helping. But there is plenty of evidence that these practices are causing anxiety, stress, trauma, morbidity and harm.

7. Too old, too fat, too Black, too risky?

A few years ago, my phone rang just as I had finished dinner.

"Hello," a voice said. *"I know you don't usually take women on late in pregnancy, but I'm 36 weeks and I really need help."*

The voice was Donna's, and she was right that I didn't usually book women in late pregnancy. Because independent midwives focus so much on relationship and the value of getting to know women and families as individuals, we like to get to know women during pregnancy. But she lived two streets away, I had a gap in my diary and, as Donna began to tell me her story, I knew that I wasn't going to say no to her.

"I'm 44," she told me. *"I had IVF and barely got that because they thought I was too fat, and I've put on quite a bit more weight in the pregnancy, despite eating healthily. I have no idea why."* Her voice broke a bit. *"My mum died when I was three months pregnant and I've had to organise all of that as well as a full-time job. I think that might be part of it…"*

I listened carefully as Donna shared more. She had seen an obstetrician that day. He told her that, because of her age, weight, and the fact that she had conceived by IVF, they would book her in for an induction on her due date. She wouldn't be allowed (he said) to give birth at home, as she had planned. When Donna had protested, the obstetrician had raised his voice, told her she was being silly and selfish, and asked her if she wanted her baby to die. Donna had walked out of the appointment in tears and she said she made a decision not to give birth in that hospital. It didn't feel safe.

At 40 weeks and 5 days, Donna gave birth on her living room floor after a six-hour labour. Her husband helped catch their baby. That baby is now a teenager with her own YouTube channel where, among other things, she talks about body confidence, self-esteem and the importance of focusing on being healthy rather than dieting.

The 'at risk' problem

I wish Donna's story of her encounter with the obstetrician was an unusual one, but it isn't. Too often, pregnant women are told that, because they are above a certain age or size, they and their baby are 'at risk' and therefore need labour induction. Women who conceived by IVF or other assisted reproductive technologies (ARTs) are also perceived to be at higher risk. And, as Donna's story shows, when women have more than one 'risk factor', the pressure to agree to induction of labour can be even greater. There are many women who are older *and* larger than average (in part because we do tend to put on weight as we age), who may be told that they are doubly or triply 'at risk,' with no good evidence.

I chose Donna's story for this chapter because she was one of the first women I cared for in this situation. The number of women offered early induction for such reasons has increased significantly since Donna gave birth. Sadly, many women and families report being pressured to agree to induction by professionals or birth workers.

"I had to fight tooth and nail to not be induced, and I'm not exaggerating. I was 45, but really healthy. Baby was healthy too. They kept referring to me as 'geriatric.' I did go into labour myself. Not at home as I had wanted, but it was alright and there weren't any problems. But the attitudes and assumptions were shocking ... if I spoke to people [in my job] *the way I was spoken to, I would be sacked."* (Libby).

"I was 'told' I was going to be induced on his due date. Not asked. I'm so grateful to him for coming early, as I didn't have the energy to fight and I don't know what I would have done. Probably just stayed home and turned the phone off. When I heard what they're planning to do to other Black women in the name of risk management, I'm incensed." (Adaobi).

Adaobi was responding to the suggestion by NICE (2021a) that induction at 39 weeks should be considered for all women who are Black, Brown, Asian or of mixed race. This proposed recommendation, as I detailed in chapter three, was greeted with considerable concern by women, midwives and birth workers. While it was true that many people have been calling for action to address the disparities experienced by Black, Brown, Asian and mixed-race people (Knight *et al* 2020), the suggestion that induction of labour should be routinely considered without good evidence of benefit came out of the blue and shocked a lot of people. The proposed recommendation was not included in the final guideline in a direct way, but the final version of the guideline (NICE 2021b) recommends that clinicians:

"Be aware that ... women from some minority ethnic backgrounds or who live in deprived areas have an increased risk of stillbirth and may need closer monitoring and additional support."

This awareness is vital. Yet the guideline does not specify what 'closer monitoring and support' might entail. Some women and professionals are worried that this may still be read as suggesting that certain groups of women should still be offered interventions, such as induction, even though we have no evidence to tell us what the effect of induction or any other intervention or monitoring would be. This is of particular concern in a context where, as I also discussed in chapter three, even an implied suggestion that something should be considered can quickly mean it becomes the norm.

When something becomes a norm, it can be particularly challenging for those who have less power, who don't understand the system, who don't speak good English or who aren't always listened to. This includes many women who are already in marginalised groups, such as refugees and asylum seekers, Black and Brown women, women who don't speak good English and those who have been trafficked or are otherwise vulnerable.

In this chapter, I'm going to look at induction for age, higher BMI and maternal race. There is so little evidence on induction in pregnancies conceived by IVF or ARTs that I can summarise what we know in a few sentences. We know that there is a higher chance of stillbirth and some other medical conditions for the mother and/or baby when pregnancy is conceived by IVF or ARTs, but there is disagreement about the exact level of increased risk (RCOG 2012b) and unfortunately we do not have good data on this. As I have written elsewhere, *"...the vast majority of babies born after IVF are born alive and well ... [and] we have no evidence about the effectiveness or safety of early labour induction."* (Wickham 2018a: 111). Decisions need to be made on an individual basis and we need more research to be carried out in this area.

The downsides of looking at single factors

I'm not a fan of putting people into boxes and categories. But, for the sake of understanding the argument, if we compare pregnant women in certain categories to pregnant women who are not in those categories then it isn't unusual to see a relative difference in risk. For example, older women are relatively more likely to experience certain kinds of problems during pregnancy and birth than younger women. Black, Brown, Asian and mixed-race women are more likely to experience problems than white women, and so on. But a few other things are also true of all these situations.

First, while there may be a relative increase in risk when we compare one group with another, the absolute chance of a complication may still remain small. Then, while it is true that women in some groups have a greater chance of a problem, it doesn't necessarily follow that intervention will reduce that chance. This is especially the case with an intervention like induction, which also carries risks of its own. It's also possible that some groups are more likely to experience problems not because they are older, larger or of a particular race, but because of the way that they are treated when they enter systems of health care. So, as we've covered elsewhere, women and families need to have good information, understand the bigger picture and, where possible, see the actual numbers, so that they can weigh up the pros and cons for themselves and make the decisions that are right for them.

Some authors are concerned about how, in research, we sometimes 'lump' groups of women together based on one characteristic, while ignoring other characteristics (Denona 2020). It's done to help us see the effect of one thing, like age or size, but it fails to take account of someone's general health. Looking at one factor (like race, weight or age) tells us very little about someone's overall health or circumstances. This is one reason why independent midwives like to get to know women and families. We get a far better sense of someone's health and wellbeing by developing a relationship over time.

Imagine, if you would, all the 40-year-old women that you know. Are they all in similar states of fitness? Of course not! Some will be gym bunnies, some won't do any exercise and some seem to take no exercise but are really fit from walking at work or super flexible from teaching yoga or looking after their kids all day. You probably know women who are vegans, vegetarians and reluctant vegetable eaters. We all know people who only ever drink at weddings and others who have barely any room for milk in their fridge door because it's so full of wine. And let's not forget those women and families who live in poverty who have nothing in their fridge, can't access a healthy diet and couldn't afford to even think about going to a gym. There is a huge link between poverty, health and size and we also know that women who live in poverty don't get good maternity care (Nagahawatte & Goldenberg 2008, Heys *et al* 2021). More on that below.

Not that any of these things are an absolute reflection of health on their own, and fitness is only one aspect of physical health. Ever met a ninety-year-old smoker who doesn't believe cigarettes are harmful because, well, it never hurt them? Just because something is known to be health-promoting, health-reducing or a risk factor on a population basis doesn't mean that it will be an issue for everyone. The research findings are true, in that they tell us what is healthy and less healthy on a *population* basis. But we're all individuals and, with apologies for the repetition, individuals vary.

What about factors such as stress levels, social life, self-esteem and community involvement? The way people see themselves and are treated by and connected with others can have a big impact. And these things are all interconnected. Looking at single factors – and here we're seeing the effects of reductionism again – means we miss the bigger picture of someone's overall health and wellbeing. Population risk data cannot predict whether or not you will personally experience a particular outcome. To some extent, as Libby said, you can assess whether you are healthy in general. It's true that, depending on your and your baby's health and situation, the risks and benefits of something can look quite different. But no matter how many factors we take into account, risk is just another word for chance. There's no way to get a guarantee, regardless of whether or not you choose a particular intervention. We're back to, 'it's complicated'.

What also complicates things is that, just like with the post-term situation, some of these recommendations to accept induction are based on research that is older, and was carried out at a time when practice and knowledge was different, so the results don't necessarily still apply today. Another issue is that some women, like Donna, have two or more 'risk factors.' More than one woman in this situation has told me that listening to professionals made them feel as if they were, *"…almost a walking time bomb."* I frequently hear from women who have been given lists of reasons why their labour should be induced. Often, there is no evidence to show that induction is beneficial for any of the reasons, but when several so-called 'risk factors' are listed in the same breath, it sounds scary. Some people might think it's plausible that, if one falls into several categories where risk is slightly increased, that this compounds their risk. But we don't know if that's true or not. And in many cases of mixed risk factors, the absolute risk still remains small, and the intervention itself still carries risks of its own. There still might not be any benefit to early induction.

But let's look at the actual evidence in each of these three areas – age, size, and ancestry.

Older women, induction and risk

While there is some evidence that older women may be more likely to have a stillbirth compared to younger women (Huang *et al* 2008, Pasupathy *et al* 2011, Knight *et al* 2017), there are a few things to know about the quality of the data on which this is based. For example, Huang *et al* (2008) carried out a systematic review and meta-analysis which showed this, but the researchers noted that the magnitude of and reasons for this increased risk weren't clear and that further research was needed. It is possible that the variation in the quality of the outcome data was because the included studies were really varied in design. The research problems that I discussed in chapter four also occur in the research on stillbirth and maternal age. For example, some studies were recent and some were twenty years old. Some included only healthy women and some included women with pre-existing illnesses or medical conditions that developed in pregnancy. There was no consensus as to what the cut-off point for 'advanced maternal age' was. The studies also defined stillbirth itself differently, in that they used different cut-off gestational ages (Wickham 2016). One key thing that we can see from the data in this review is that, contrary to what some women are told, the risk does not suddenly dramatically increase once someone passes their 35th birthday. This is another situation where there is no 'pumpkin moment.' In reality, the risk increases a bit each year, but it is also dependent on someone's general health.

Huang *et al* (2008) did show that at least some of the increased risk is due to age alone. But healthy older women need to be aware that the data on risk are for the whole population of older pregnant women, which includes women with medical conditions that might in themselves increase the chance of an adverse outcome. It is possible that, if we looked only at healthy women, there wouldn't be as much of a difference. When this has been attempted though, the only way of getting large enough numbers is to include studies that are decades old. As we saw in chapter four, this isn't ideal either. Many things have changed over time, and initiatives have been put in place which would likely prevent some of the stillbirths that occurred in those early studies from occurring nowadays.

In 2016, a randomised controlled trial was carried out to evaluate the effect of early induction of labour at 39 weeks in older women (Walker *et al* 2016a). This study has been termed the '35/39 trial,' as it defined older women as those aged 35 and above. However, although many people thought that this study was going to compare stillbirth rates, not enough women agreed to enter the trial to be able to do that.

As with the later ARRIVE trial which I discussed in chapter five, 86% of the women who were asked to participate in the 35/39 trial declined. Only 619 women were randomised into the study; a small number on which to base recommendations. This may again reflect women's reluctance to have induction or to have the mode of onset of their labour determined by chance. In fact, the researchers noted that, *"Among the 46% of eligible nonparticipants who expressed a preference for one of the management strategies, 1595 of 1804 women (88%) preferred expectant management."* (Walker *et al* 2016a). This again confirms that many women prefer labour not to be induced and also that those women who do agree to participate in studies such as the 35/39 trial are more likely to be in favour of induction. This means that, when any qualitative research is done alongside these quantitative studies, the results are fairly meaningless because the women who agree to participate in such trials aren't representative of the general population; they are more likely to favour or at least not mind the idea of early induction. So the fact that there were no significant differences in these women's experiences is unsurprising.

There were no maternal or neonatal deaths in either group and no differences in the frequency of adverse outcomes, which also isn't surprising in such a small study. As with some other induction studies, the data from the 35/39 trial showed no difference in caesarean section rates between the two groups. Additionally, the 35/39 trial suffered some of the same limitations as the ARRIVE trial, which I also discussed in chapter five. For example, even some of the proponents of offering routine induction to older women acknowledge that professional decision making is a key factor affecting the caesarean rate (RCOG 2013). Other studies have confirmed that, compared to younger women, older women are more likely to end up with a caesarean if their labour is induced (Ankarcrona *et al* 2019) and that there is a lower threshold for caesareans in older women (Wang *et al* 2011, Carolan *et al* 2011). The chance of caesarean is even higher when it is a woman's first baby. Scandinavian researchers calculated that, *"The absolute risk of cesarean section is 3-5 times higher across 5-year age groups in nulliparous relative to multiparous women having induced labor."* (Bergholt *et al* 2020).

In simple terms, when caregivers become worried that being older is a risk factor, they suggest intervention sooner. The intervention itself can lead to negative consequences, such as increased bleeding, and a self-fulfilling prophecy is created. We can then never work out how many (if any) of the unwanted consequences were genuinely the result of older age, and how many were the result of the extra interventions which were offered because a practitioner was fearful about whether being older might put someone more at risk.

The next key study on early induction in older women was published by Knight *et al* (2017). This was a large study of data from 77,327 first-time mothers aged 35 or older who gave birth in NHS hospitals in England. It was not a randomised controlled trial, which is the best way to test the short-term outcomes of an intervention such as induction but, as we have seen, these are difficult to carry out. In this cohort study, there was no difference in perinatal mortality with induction at 39 weeks compared to waiting. There did seem to be a difference in perinatal mortality at 40 weeks, although the researchers calculated that 562 inductions would have to be carried out in order to prevent one perinatal death. When one considers the potentially serious risks, downsides and long-term effects of induction on maternal and child health (which is discussed in chapter one), that does seem a concerningly large number of mothers and babies to expose to unnecessary induction.

A study from The Netherlands has given us the most recent data on the actual risk figures. Unfortunately, the researchers used large blocks to describe age-related risk and, as I've already said, risk increases gradually over time and not steeply after big birthdays. But these are the best and most recent data that we have. Kortekaas *et al* (2020) looked at women in three different age groups; 18-35, 35-39 and 40 and above. They used something called a composite perinatal outcome, which includes minor conditions or observed outcomes that don't affect long-term health as well as more major adverse outcomes. I have shared their key findings below, expressed in terms of the actual (absolute) chance of a problem and not the relative chance. Looking at relative risk is generally really unhelpful. It can often make things sound more likely than they really are. Also, if you're 39, it's not as if you can jump in the TARDIS and reduce your age to one with a lower risk score by going back in time a few years. People need to know the numbers for where they're at.

In Kortekass *et al*'s (2020) study, the chance of neonatal death was the same across all age groups, but the stillbirth rate was different depending on maternal age.

Women in the 18-35 age group had a 0.17 chance of stillbirth, which is 1 in 588.
Women in the 35-39 age group had a 0.22 chance of stillbirth, which is 1 in 455.
Women in the 40+ age group had a 0.30 chance of stillbirth, which is 1 in 333.

Overall, Kortekass *et al* (2020) found that both advancing maternal age (AMA) and increasing gestational age increased the chance of a problem. Interestingly, *"…the association between gestational age and composite adverse perinatal and maternal outcomes was slightly stronger than the association with AMA."* (Kortekaas *et al* 2020: 1022). In other words, being older is less of a risk factor than going far beyond your due date, and we've already looked at that in chapter five and seen that the risk isn't as great as people think. In this study, *"… the absolute risk of a serious event remains low and the differences between the different age groups are small."* (Kortekaas *et al* 2020: 1022).

Maternal age: the wider issues

I want to add a few quick points here about the wider issues relating to maternal age. It's easy to overlook these things when we focus solely on short-term outcomes. One is that, as with some other areas, there is evidence that outcomes for older women are better if they have midwifery care and, for healthy women, if they birth outside of a hospital (Li *et al* 2014). Another important consideration is that, when it comes to advanced maternal age, most stillbirths are explained by congenital abnormalities (Walker *et al* 2016b, Kortekaas *et al* 2020). Some of the studies that I have discussed in this section have controlled for that. But sadly, inducing labour won't prevent all of those deaths, or make babies better.

There are important questions to be asked about the routine offer of induction in older mothers. Pasupathy *et al*'s (2011) study concluded that the increase they found in stillbirths in women aged 40 or over was the result of hypoxia in labour, which means a reduction in the amount of oxygen that the baby received in labour. If this is the case, it is hard to see how routine induction of labour can be justified as an appropriate response. Induction of labour generally involves the use of synthetic oxytocin, and one of the many downsides of using synthetic oxytocin is that it can cause hypoxia (Buckley 2015, Wickham 2016).

I want to finish this section with an important reminder. *"Research reports and recommendations… tend to ignore the positive aspects of advancing maternal age. These include the likelihood that psychological and social strengths, such as increased confidence, may more than compensate for any biological problems with which advanced age may be associated."* (Mander 2013: 49). There are advantages to being an older parent, and when we focus only on the possible downsides, we miss seeing that.

Understanding the importance of disadvantage

Before I look at the issues relating to larger women and Black and Brown women, I want to raise some issues which are significant in both of these situations and others. Many women are disadvantaged, for many different reasons, and often for more than one reason. Poverty, social disadvantage and the prejudice and poor care that often accompanies this is a significant problem. We also need to be aware of the additional burdens experienced by pregnant women who are poor, single, homeless, trafficked, refugees, travellers, prisoners or from other disadvantaged and vulnerable groups. These women experience worse maternal outcomes and have a greater chance of their baby dying (Knight *et al* 2018). Black, Brown, Asian and mixed-race women face the additional burdens of microaggressions, weathering (which I will discuss below) and institutional and systemic racism (Giscombe & Lobel 2005, Muglu *et al* 2019, Knight *et al* 2018, 2020, Lokugamage *et al* 2021).

We are only just beginning to unpack the issues and links between some of these disadvantages, for instance how poverty can be linked with ill health and higher BMI in some women. Disadvantages and vulnerabilities are often complex and inter-related and many women face other prejudices, including sexism, ageism and sizeism.

As a recent study has shown, "[disadvantaged] ...*women's vulnerability was compounded by complex life factors, judgmental and stigmatizing attitudes by health professionals, and differential care provision."* (Heys *et al* 2021). The same study pointed out that, *"Continuity of midwifery care could enhance relationship based individualised care for disadvantaged and vulnerable women."* (Heys *et al* 2021). Other research has confirmed that continuity of midwifery care can be particularly helpful for disadvantaged women (Sandall *et al* 2016, Homer *et al* 2017).

It's really clear that there is a lot of work to be done, and that offering routine intervention rather than individualised care is a poor response to a complex problem that affects many people. I will return to this later in the book, but I mention it now because disadvantage is a key issue for some of the women in the groups that I will discuss in the remainder of this chapter: those with a higher BMI and those who are Black, Brown, Asian or of mixed race.

What about larger women?

Larger women are often told about research which shows that they are more likely to have a stillborn baby compared to women of average size (Flenady *et al* 2011, Woolner & Bhattacharya 2015, Denison *et al* 2018). They aren't always told that there is some debate about this, or that there is no evidence that induction improves outcomes for the babies born to larger women. They may also not be told that, just like older women, larger women are not a homogeneous group, and that individual health and wellbeing may be a more significant factor than size alone.

BMI (or body mass index, which is the most common way of measuring how large someone is within a western medical framework) is considered a very crude measuring tool. There's very little evidence showing that the current approach to weight and size taken by western medicine is helping anyone, least of all larger people. We know that larger women are at risk of weight stigma in maternity care – which is just one form of the disadvantage that I described in the previous section – and that the wider health services are getting things very wrong when it comes to attitudes to and the information shared with larger people (Kerrigan *et al* 2015, Knight-Agarwal *et al* 2016, Treasure & Ambwani 2021). There isn't any evidence that losing weight actually improves the health of people with higher BMI (Woolner & Bhattacharya 2015, Treasure & Ambwani 2021, Wolrich 2021). Many larger women report experiencing weight stigma and stereotyping (Knight-Agarwal *et al* 2016, Jones & Jomeen 2017, Relph *et al* 2020) and being given inaccurate information about risk.

"It was drilled into me by consultant after consultant that because my BMI was higher I would almost certainly have a stillborn baby if I allowed the pregnancy to go past 39 weeks. I was devastated and terrified so I agreed to a induction. I was admitted at 40 weeks and was still sat on the induction ward at 41 weeks. My induction began after 6 hours but I had to wait day after day for a labour ward bed. Ultimately it all ended in a traumatising c section. I will never have another induction." (Antonia).

One of the most serious concerns about this area is that, although organisations such as the RCOG recommend that, *"…obese pregnant women should be made aware that they are at increased risk of stillbirth"* (Denison *et al* 2018), this recommendation is based on 'level D' evidence, which is considered to be low grade. Some of the reviews that have been carried out (e.g. Aune *et al* 2014) include data from countries with high perinatal mortality rates, and also include babies who were lost early in pregnancy, which makes outcomes look worse than they are in reality, especially for those in high-income countries. Some of the papers looking at stillbirth in larger women cite an increased risk on a relative basis but do not give the raw data, which means that we can't calculate the absolute chance of stillbirth in different groups. This is frustrating, because if someone says that something is twice as likely to happen, they might mean that the risk has gone from one in ten to one in five, or they might mean that the risk has gone from one in two million to one in a million. Those are very different sets of numbers, which is why we need to know the absolute chance of something happening as well. But those data aren't available.

Induction outcomes in larger women

There are no randomised controlled trials that have looked at outcomes relating to larger women and induction of labour. So we don't have any robust evidence to tell us whether or not induction is beneficial for larger women or their babies. Some researchers are calling for randomised controlled trials to look at induction in larger women (Coates *et al* 2020b, D'Souza *et al* 2021). Given the problems in the trials that have looked at induction for post-term pregnancy, suspected macrosomia and older maternal age, however, it is difficult to be sure that any trial looking at induction for larger women would tell us anything except that this group of women are also more likely to be told they need a caesarean, whether or not this is the case by any objective measure.

We do have some data from retrospective studies, which look back at women's medical records to see what happened in different groups of women, but the results are very mixed and not very reliable. In some hospitals, larger women who had induction were less likely to be told they needed a caesarean than women who received expectant management (Lee *et al* 2016, Glazer *et al* 2020). But in others the chance of caesarean was the same for larger women no matter whether labour was spontaneous or induced (Kawakita *et al* 2017). Several studies found that induction increases the chance of caesarean in larger women (Wolfe *et al* 2014, Ruhstaller 2015, Little *et al* 2019, Carlhäll *et al* 2020, Hamm *et al* 2021).

Most of the studies show no difference in outcomes or do not look at this. The results of those that do show a difference vary. Pickens *et al* (2018) found fewer adverse outcomes in babies born to larger women who had induction. By contrast, Wolfe *et al* (2014) found that the babies born to larger women (with a BMI of 30 or more) whose labours were induced were more likely to be admitted to neonatal intensive care. It's very difficult to draw any conclusions when the results vary so much between studies. We should also bear in mind that all larger women are at risk of being told they need intervention in mainstream maternity care. In Dalbye *et al*'s (2021) study, larger women in spontaneous labour were more likely to be told that they needed a caesarean or that their labour needed to be augmented, or speeded up with drugs. In addition, as with many of the studies that I have discussed in previous chapters, most of these studies are American and are based on a very medicalised approach to birth. The samples aren't representative of larger women in general and, again, outcomes are affected by professional decisions.

Taking a woman-centred view

There is good reason to question the idea that induction might be beneficial for larger women and there is also evidence for the idea that we should take a different view about the care of women with a higher BMI.

In a Norwegian study of healthy women who gave birth to a single, head-down baby at term between 2014 and 2017, there were no differences in neonatal outcomes for women of different sizes (Dalbye *et al* 2021). And Relph *et al* (2021) showed that, *"...over half of women with obesity but no other preexisting medical or early obstetric complicating factors, proceed through pregnancy without adverse obstetric complication."*

In the UK, a study called the UKMidSS Severe Obesity Study (Rowe *et al* 2018) gave us some important information about larger women who gave birth in alongside midwifery units (AMUs). This was a prospective cohort study using the UK Midwifery Study System (UKMidSS) and data were collected from all of the 122 AMUs in the UK at the time. The outcomes of larger women were compared with the outcomes of women with a BMI under 35.

The researchers found that, for the women having their second or later baby), *"...the severely obese group [women with a BMI of between 35 and 40kg/m2] were no more likely than other multiparous women admitted to AMUs to experience an obstetric intervention or adverse maternal outcome, after adjustment for maternal characteristics, and almost all (96%) had a 'straight-*

forward vaginal birth'. We found no evidence of increased risk in any adverse maternal or perinatal outcomes, compared with other multiparous women admitted to AMUs." (Rowe *et al* 2018).

The chance of a problem was slightly higher for women having their first baby, and the researchers,

"…found that the severely obese group had a non-significant 14% increased risk of experiencing an obstetric intervention or adverse maternal outcome, but our analysis was underpowered to detect a difference of this magnitude as statistically significant." (Rowe *et al* 2018).

Of the 'severely obese' women having their first baby, 67.9% had a straightforward vaginal birth. The point is that, even if there is a slightly higher chance that intervention will be needed and that larger woman having their first baby will experience an adverse outcome such as higher blood loss after the birth, most larger women and their babies don't need intervention or experience an adverse outcome and they may be more likely to have a good outcome if they are cared for in a midwifery-led setting.

Some health professionals are working hard to take a more holistic, individualised approach to the care of larger women (Kerrigan *et al* 2015). Midwives who work closely with women and form trusting relationships with them (such as Donna, whose story I shared above) often report that they do not see increased caesarean section rates or poorer outcomes in larger women. Another recent study confirmed that larger women who were cared for by midwives had far fewer caesareans and fewer tears than women cared for by obstetricians. The women were also significantly less likely to have oxytocin and some other interventions and more likely to move around, use birthing pools and to have intermittent rather than continuous fetal monitoring in labour. All other maternal and neonatal outcomes were equal in both groups (Carlson *et al* 2017). And in a study of larger women who gave birth in birth centres:

"The majority of women with obese BMIs experienced uncomplicated perinatal courses and vaginal births. There were no

significant differences in antenatal complications, proportion of prolonged pregnancy, prolonged first and second stage labor, rupture of membranes longer than 24 hours, postpartum hemorrhage, or newborn outcomes between women with obese BMIs and normal BMIs... Women with obese BMIs without medical comorbidity can receive safe and effective midwifery care at freestanding birth centers while anticipating a low risk for cesarean birth. The risks of potential, obesity-related perinatal complications should be discussed with women when choosing place of birth; however, pregnancy complicated by obesity must be viewed holistically, not simply through the lens of obesity." (Jevitt *et al* 2021: 14).

BMI and size: other considerations

There are some other issues to consider when it comes to the care offered to larger women. Larger women are more likely than average-sized women to be told they need a caesarean, no matter how their labour begins (Bergholt *et al* 2007, Zhang *et al* 2007, Kominariak *et al* 2010, Fyfe *et al* 2011, Crequit *et al* 2020). However, this may be partly or wholly due to care provider attitudes rather than simply the consequence of factors relating to the woman or her size.

Larger women's wombs are said to contract less efficiently than those of average-sized women (Zhang *et al* 2007). Research has not adequately tested this theory, so it's impossible to know whether there is any truth to this or whether it's another myth that is wholly or partially rooted in attitudes to women, and to larger women in particular.

Some research shows that some larger women may have longer labours (Carlhäll *et al* 2020), which may lead to care provider impatience or a higher chance of the baby becoming distressed. But it is incredibly difficult to tease out the factors that affect length of labour, as this is influenced by the environment (including the attitudes and actions of the people within it) as well as factors to do with the woman, baby and labour. As most of the research that we have has been carried out in hospitals, we have very little evidence about outcomes of women and babies who receive more holistic and individualised care, and whose labours progress physiologically (Edwards 2019).

As I noted in chapter four, larger women are more likely to end up with an inaccurate due date if scans are used to date pregnancy (Källén *et al* 2013, Kullinger *et al* 2016). Ironically, though, guidelines tend to recommend more ultrasounds in larger women because of concerns that manual measurement and estimation of fetal size may be less accurate in larger women (Denison *et al* 2018). We don't know how many of the challenges experienced by larger women are the result of having more scans or scan-related errors. It's also possible that the small number of women whose babies would genuinely benefit from induction are not being offered this at an appropriate time because of the inaccuracy of ultrasound due date estimation.

Researchers, guidelines and practitioners also continue to recommend weight loss, despite the fact that dieting has been shown to be an ineffective strategy for long-term weight loss and there is no evidence that thinness equates with health or that higher weight equates with poor health (Treasure & Ambwani 2021, Wolrich 2021). There is also no evidence that dieting (at any stage of life – not just during pregnancy) is safe or beneficial (Woolner & Bhattacharya 2015). Evidence is emerging about how factors such as stress and the number and type of bacteria that someone has in their gut may affect their weight more than what they eat or how much they exercise (Duan *et al* 2021).

But this knowledge isn't making much difference in practice. Weight stigma in health care and in society in general is a significant problem (Relph *et al* 2020, Iacobucci 2020, Treasure & Ambwani 2021, Wolrich 2021) and the recommendation to offer induction of labour to larger women may be the result of this. People avoid medical care because of it, which may partly explain why there is an increased chance of unwanted outcomes. Stigma can also be seen among obesity researchers (Flint & Reale 2014) and even some of the papers that have sought women's views still talk about weight 'management,' which is only one possible approach. This highlights the disadvantage faced by larger women, which is exacerbated when the same women are also disadvantaged because of being poor, Black, Brown, Asian or mixed-race, a refugee or asylum seeker, a non-English speaker or any of the factors that I described above.

It is possible that the same things that are causing some people to weigh more are also affecting their babies. As I've already noted, poverty, vulnerability and social disadvantage are key factors for some women. Where women are poor, vulnerable, disadvantaged and/or living with high levels of stress, treating symptoms such as higher BMI won't remove the problem. Again, we need to move away from a reductionist approach and find better ways of thinking about the situation that our society faces. Poverty doesn't affect every woman who is larger than average, but it is a factor for some. We should not be making recommendations based on single factors. We must look at women as individuals and offer the kind of care that has been shown to make a positive difference. Good midwifery care cannot reduce inequalities, but it can ameliorate their impacts (Nadine Edwards, personal correspondence 2021).

Given that larger women are more at risk of a range of negative consequences if they undergo induction of labour, and as caesarean carries more risk for larger women than for women of average size, it may be more appropriate (and less risky) to promote midwifery care and some of these other ways of helping larger women to avoid unnecessary induction. These approaches include ensuring that women have non-judgemental care providers, can birth in out-of-hospital settings if this is their preference and are not subjected to routine appointments and assessments in which practitioners and health service employees seek to shame them for being larger and cast doubt on their ability to grow a healthy baby and give birth. Women need to be able to mobilise in labour and access tools that promote physiological birth, such as the use of water during labour and birth.

Sadly, some hospitals tell larger women that they may not access such facilities, Sometimes they claim that larger women need to be on a consultant unit rather than a midwifery-led birth centre because there isn't suitable equipment, or that it is too hard to help women out of a pool if difficulties arise. This not only denies women choice. It also denies women the tools and environments that give them the best chance of a successful physiological labour and birth. Such an approach increases the chance of further intervention and makes it more likely that larger women and their babies will experience the negative consequences of this.

In summary, when it comes to maternal size, the lack of evidence to support the idea of intervention, the degree of uncertainty and the complexity of the issues mean that a population level recommendation for induction could do more harm than good. It would be far better to offer women respectful, individualised, supportive midwifery care which is not based on outdated and unevidenced ideas about size.

Maternal race, racism and induction

It is very clear that Black, Brown, Asian and mixed-race women are at risk of adverse outcomes for both themselves and their babies when they give birth in systems of care designed by and for white people (Giscombe & Lobel 2005, Muglu *et al* 2019, Knight *et al* 2020, Lokugamage *et al* 2021). Wherever white women are oppressed in systems of health care, Black and Brown women fare even worse. There is abundant evidence of this, and of wider health inequalities and disparities which researchers have long attributed to systemic racism (Giscombe & Lobel 2005, Anekwe 2020, Knight *et al* 2020, Marmot *et al* 2020, Razai *et al* 2021).

The suggestion that practitioners should consider early induction in Black, Brown, Asian and mixed-race women was included in the draft NICE (2021a) guideline without precedent or warning, so I have included this section in my book as a brief overview, but with the caveat that I am not an expert in this field and it needs far more attention.

We have significant evidence of racism within the systems of care where induction is offered (Knight *et al* 2020, Marmot *et al* 2020, Lokugamage *et al* 2021). We know that we need to dismantle some of the systems and structures that are negatively affecting all women, and this is particularly important when it comes to racism and racial inequalities. That applies both within maternity care and more widely. But we know very little about whether or how racism and its consequences affect the length of pregnancy and the onset of labour. We also know that poverty, vulnerability and social disadvantage, as well as the issues that stem from these, disproportionately affect Black, Brown, Asian and mixed-race women, which adds to the constellation of problems and biases that some woman face.

As with older women and larger women, we know that Black, Brown, Asian and mixed-race women experience higher rates of perinatal mortality. Muglu *et al* (2019) found abundant evidence that health care systems are failing Black mothers and babies. Black mothers are one and a half to two times more likely to lose a baby during every week of pregnancy compared to white women. But there is no evidence that routine early induction improves outcomes in Black, Brown, Asian and mixed-race women. No studies have been done that can tell us this; not one.

Importantly, not only does induction have risks and long-term consequences, but it is possible that these may be greater in women who are already at a disadvantage. And, for all these reasons, we particularly need to ensure that a more individualised, culturally safe, person-centred approach is taken to the health and maternity care of Black, Brown, Asian and mixed-race women.

Ancestral variation and weathering

As I mentioned in chapter four, I have concern about how some people are interpreting the data showing that Black and Asian women tend to give birth earlier than white women. I am not denying that studies have found this, in Black women (Papiernik *et al* 1990, Mittendorf *et al* 1993, Omigbodun & Adewuyi 1997, Patel *et al* 2003) and Asian women (Khambalia *et al* 2013). Anecdotally, this has also been observed by midwives and doctors. But we cannot draw any conclusions from these results, and there are several reasons for this.

Some of the early studies used racist language, which gives us a clue about the lens through which the researchers were working. Others focused primarily on white women and did not include enough Black women to determine whether any difference was genuine. Any differences seen in such studies are generally small. In Khambalia *et al*'s (2013) study, which is probably the most robust of those I cited, the difference in the average length of pregnancy between Asian and white Australian women was only three days. Another concern is that data on race are often poorly recorded in medical records and research (Knight *et al* 2020). This means that we cannot be sure that we are counting the right women in the right groups. And, of course, data on groups can only tell us about groups, or populations, not about individuals.

"In the NICE evidence review for the draft guidelines the lack of direct evidence for women from ethnic minorities is noted by NICE. Of the studies referenced the vast majority did not record race or were unable to, or failed to, report on ethnic variation due to low numbers of minority ethnic women. This "absence" of evidence could be construed as a form of structural racism." (Douglass & Lokugamage 2021).

But even if Black and/or Asian women do experience comparatively shorter pregnancies, we have no evidence that this is problematic or that offering induction of labour will be of any benefit. Moreover, even if there is a genuine difference in the length of labour between Black, Asian and white populations, we cannot know whether it is a genetically based difference between groups of people with different ancestry, the result of research bias, poverty, social disadvantage, weathering or several of those things and perhaps others.

The weathering hypothesis was first proposed by Geronimus (1992), who was trying to explain the different outcomes between African American and non-Hispanic white mothers and infants. It describes the idea that *"...the health of African-American women may begin to deteriorate in early adulthood as a physical consequence of cumulative socioeconomic disadvantage."* (Geronimus 1992: 207). Another way of putting this is that the constant stress of racism and the disadvantages that it brings can lead to premature biological aging and other poorer health outcomes (Simons *et al* 2016, Cerdeña *et al* 2020, Lokugamage *et al* 2021). It's also possible that poor health due to disadvantage can result in shorter pregnancies, but we just don't know. If weathering is the reason that Black and Asian women have a tendency towards shorter pregnancies, then this is, again, not evidence *for* intervention but evidence *of* racism. As Douglass and Lokugamage (2021) also point out, *"...NICE ... has, within its new draft guidelines for induction of labour, a suggestion of racial profiling."*

Offering earlier induction to Black and Brown women could have a very negative effect. As I discussed in chapter one, we know that induction leads to an increase in interventions, which carry risks. This is not advantageous to women and babies who are already at higher risk of dying in childbirth because of the effects of racism, poverty and social disadvantage (Knight *et al* 2020). In addition, as Douglass and Lokugamage (2021) pointed out in their response to the draft NICE guidance:

"We are deeply concerned that if these recommendations are taken forward uncritically, they could further embed institutional racism in maternity care, strengthen racial biases and stereotypes, legitimise skin tone as clinically meaningful, pathologize healthy pregnancies in women from ethnic minority backgrounds, and undermine choice for black and brown women." (Douglass & Lokugamage 2021).

Routine induction isn't the answer

As I have stated many times now, population trends can't tell us anything about individuals, and it is impossible to separate out different factors that can impact outcomes. This means that we need to analyse the issues carefully before recommending interventions that could make things worse. Even suggesting that clinicians consider offering early induction of labour is not only an inappropriate response to the fact that Black, Brown, Asian and mixed-race women and babies have poorer outcomes than their white counterparts. It's incredibly disappointing given the recent focus on raising awareness about how Black and Brown women have been abused in the name of medicine and science. Anecdotally, some activists have described the recent push towards considering offering early induction to Black, Brown, Asian and mixed-race women as racist.

We need to understand that at least some (and perhaps a lot) of the disadvantage faced by Black, Brown, Asian and mixed-race women comes about through stress and other social, environmental and systemic factors and consider how to address this. The first things we need to address relate to reducing stress and the negative impact of poverty and social disadvantage.

I have discussed midwife-led care and how this can make a positive difference in several of the situations in which induction is routinely offered (Sandall *et al* 2016, Homer *et al* 2017). When it comes to race, the outcomes of the Albany midwifery practice demonstrate that poorer outcomes for Black and Brown people are not an inevitability. In research into the Albany midwifery model, 57% of the women whose data were included in this study were from Black, Brown and Asian communities, and the data from this study show that good midwifery care can make even more of a positive difference to these women (Homer *et al* 2017). Making good midwifery care a reality for all women and families would require commitment, change and a willingness on the part of those who hold the power and who benefit from the current system to accept that we're not currently getting it right.

But the bottom line for those concerned about being offered induction for maternal race is that there is no evidence to suggest that it would be beneficial. It may be that the proposed recommendation was a response to the data showing that Black, Brown., Asian and mixed-race women and their babies have a higher chance of poorer outcomes compared to white women and their babies. But induction of labour is not an appropriate answer to systemic racism, especially without any evidence of benefit.

To return to the other issues discussed in this chapter, evidence does not support the idea that routine early induction of labour is the answer for older or larger women either. It's really clear that we need a different approach, and I will consider that in the final chapter of this book.

8. Addressing the induction epidemic

"Most women prefer giving birth without interventions and value having a positive childbirth experience in addition to healthy outcomes (Downe et al 2018). Induction of labour often results in a cascade of interventions that are neither pleasant nor empowering for women. Minimising obstetric interventions and giving support to childbearing women improves maternal experiences of childbirth and enhances empowerment. Offering induction to all women at term ignores the principles of the Hippocratic oath, 'first, do no harm' and should therefore only be reserved for women with a clear medical indication." (Seijmonsbergen-Schermers *et al* 2019).

When the 2008 version of the NICE induction of labour guideline was published, one in five women had their labour induced (NICE 2008a). We know that, during the pandemic, the average induction rate in the UK Trusts and Health Boards that responded in one study was 34%, which is one in three women (Harkness *et al* 2021). The rates in other high-income countries are similar, and in some cases higher. As I was writing this book, some colleagues shared with me that the rate in their area is nearing 50%, or one in two women.

But the evidence for offering induction to this many women is lacking. As many of the researchers that I have cited in this book have concluded, spontaneous labour confers many advantages and should be the default option: induction has short-, medium- and long-term downsides for women, babies and families. In this book, I have tried to explain this evidence as well as to tell the story of how we have ended up in this situation. I have also explained that induction can be very helpful in some situations. If a woman or baby has a medical condition, the benefits of earlier birth may outweigh the risk of being born too early and the negative consequences of the interventions involved in induction. But, in most situations, evidence shows that induction isn't beneficial just because someone has a risk factor.

It's clear that we need changes to the way we approach

pregnancy, birth and induction of labour. This recent summary of the evidence for routine induction in different situations summarises the difference between the evidence and the current guidelines:

"Available evidence supports IOL for women with post-term pregnancy, although the evidence is weak regarding the timing (41 versus 42 weeks), and for women with hypertension/preeclampsia in terms of improved maternal outcomes. For women with preterm premature [prelabour] *rupture of membranes (24–37 weeks), high-quality evidence supports expectant management rather than IOL/early birth. Evidence is weakly supportive for IOL in women with term rupture of membranes. For all other indications, there were conflicting findings and/or insufficient power to provide definitive evidence."* (Coates *et al* 2020b).

But many women and families don't know this and aren't being given accurate information about the evidence about medical interventions such as induction. Most are persuaded into taking a medicalised path, and those who question this are sometimes subjected to coercion, frightening them into complying with the medical norm. As in other areas of life, people who challenge the status quo, including the midwives, doctors and others who are battling for change, may find themselves bullied, belittled and scorned by people who believe strongly in the medical model.

Solutions that aren't helping

It's important to bear in mind that some of the things that people think are the answer to the induction epidemic are in themselves problematic. Offering women routine membrane sweeping at 38 or 39 weeks is not a solution or an alternative to induction of labour. It is in itself a form of induction. Membrane sweeping undermines women's trust in their own bodies and rhythms. It ignores the benefits of going into spontaneous labour and, if it does work, it could bring labour on too soon for some babies. In many cases, it doesn't work. In some cases, the midwife or doctor performing the membrane sweep will accidentally break the waters, which means there is a greater chance of infection, so medical intervention may be offered and the woman will then have to make decisions that she wouldn't have faced if she hadn't had a membrane sweep. Membrane sweeping is uncomfortable or traumatic for some women. See my website (Wickham 2020) for more information on this.

Another option that isn't the answer to the induction epidemic is ironically adding to the increased caesarean rate. This is because some people are wondering if planned caesarean is a better alternative to induction.

"I really don't want to have induction if I go overdue. Everyone I know who has one has a horrible, lonely experience in the hospital for days on end and then ends up with a caesarean section anyway. Why don't they just be honest and give us the option of a section in the first place?" (Freda).

"I've started to suggest to women that, if they don't want induction, they can ask for a planned caesarean instead. I think it's less traumatic for them." (Kelly, doula).

Like induction, planned caesarean can be useful if the woman or baby has a medical condition in which the benefits outweigh the risks. But it carries many of the same risks as induction, including the baby possibly being born too soon and the risks and side effects of the drugs used. It's true that caesarean is a relatively safe operation nowadays, but it is still less safe than having a physiological labour and birth.

"[Caesarean section] *is associated with an increased risk of uterine rupture, abnormal placentation, ectopic pregnancy, stillbirth, and preterm birth, and these risks increase in a dose–response manner. There is emerging evidence that babies born by CS have different hormonal, physical, bacterial, and medical exposures, and that these exposures can subtly alter neonatal physiology. Short-term risks of CS include altered immune development, an increased likelihood of allergy, atopy, and asthma, and reduced intestinal gut microbiome diversity. The persistence of these risks into later life is less well investigated, although an association between CS use and greater incidence of late childhood obesity and asthma are frequently reported."* (Sandall *et al* 2018: 1349).

Caesarean can be particularly problematic for some groups of women. For instance, planned caesarean has a higher chance of complications for older women and researchers suggest that surgery should be avoided in older women unless truly essential (Lavecchia *et al* 2018). Surgery is also well known to carry more risk for larger people.

At the other end of the spectrum, fear of induction, other intervention, coercion and disrespectful treatment can lead some women to avoid the maternity services altogether and freebirth, which means to give birth without a qualified birth attendant such as a midwife or doctor. If freebirth is a genuine preference, then that's one thing. But no woman should have to opt for something they don't really want, to settle for a plan B because a reasonable request isn't being met or the only thing that's being offered within the maternity services is unacceptable to them. If you are finding it difficult to get what you want, almost every country has people and/or organisations that support choice in maternity services. You may also want to look for a midwife who can support you, especially if you live in a country where midwifery care isn't the norm. If you are already booked for care within the maternity services, ask for a second opinion or to see a consultant midwife or a manager. Many hospitals also have patient support services and there are a wealth of resources if you search online or ask around.

What's the answer?

The answer to the problems that I have described in this book is simple, at least on paper. The answer is to move away from standardisation and to offer respectful, personalised, midwifery-led continuity of care, which has been shown in many studies to improve outcomes (Sandall *et al* 2016). We need maternity care that is woman-centred and which allows midwives to work autonomously, with obstetricians and other specialists available for those women who need and want additional medical help.

We need practitioners who understand and work with pregnancy and birth physiology. We need good childbirth education and support, including labour companionship, for all women, not just those who can afford it. We need to help those in complex situations, not blame or shame them. We need to avoid offering intervention unless truly warranted. We need to effectively address racism, agism and sizeism rather than compound these issues with policies and practices that aren't evidence based. We need to ensure that practitioners have more time to spend with women and families, so that evidence can be offered and explained in an even-handed and non-coercive way and options discussed in relation to each individual's specific circumstances which take into the account that experiences and other kinds of knowledge are more important to some people.

It's also vital to acknowledge that different approaches to research can give us distinctive but equally useful kinds of information, and that it is incredibly valuable to have diverse and varied kinds of knowledge. It is also just as important to know about women's experiences and what happens in real-world settings as it is to know what happens in the theoretical and sometimes artificial environment of a randomised controlled trial. We need more acknowledgement that study findings and real-world outcomes are affected by human decisions, and to help both the providers and recipients of health care to a better understanding of risk and evidence.

But how?

Sadly, the question of what we can do about the induction epidemic and the wider inequalities, discriminations and sometimes abuses that are embedded in maternity care is a difficult one. No one particular person, group or organisation can be challenged or called upon to change it; the values that underpin this approach are embedded in the beliefs that most of us who live in high-income countries generally accept as a beneficial part of life; most of us have accepted that it's beneficial to allow our lives to be guided by clocks and calendars without knowing how nature's rhythms affect our lives, health and bodily rhythms; and we've gained from the use of technology and some aspects of industrialisation and related systems. It is potentially beneficial to make some population recommendations or to set norms based on scientific evidence rather than on one person's experience or intuition. It's just that these ideas and approaches aren't *always* appropriate. They can sometimes be harmful and sometimes their side effects are greater than their benefits for some or most people.

Many of the tenets that I described above have been misunderstood, applied too generally and in some cases exploited by those wanting more money and power. And yet it's not as simple as saying the answer is to petition those with power. We should absolutely continue our efforts to lobby governments and the organisations that set the guidelines, and call them to account. But many have a vested interest in the status quo and, while lobbying can be effective in some situations, science, evidence and the voiced concerns of women and professionals do not always win out.

Some of the people who campaign, research or write about maternity care blame, petition and call for midwives and doctors to change their ways and practise differently. Their discussion and conclusions often include the words, *'Midwives should…'* or *'Doctors should…'* and then go on to exhort professionals to change their ways.

I'm not going to argue that all professionals and birth workers are angels or that they aren't part of the problem, because that's not true. There are things that anyone who works with women and families can do to improve their own practice and approach and to highlight issues in their place of work. But midwives and doctors are far more constrained than many people realise. Health professionals are workers in a system run by corporations, which operate according to the capitalist, patriarchal values that I described in chapter two. This is why systems of health care are rife with sexism, racism, classism and ableism, to name but a few of the problems.

Mavis Kirkham explains how the economic and political context in which midwives and doctors work and the pressure that is put on them often means that they barely have time to give the most basic care, let alone ensure that women and families receive the information they need:

"There is a great deal of 'midwives should' writing and it is added to daily in books, articles and theses. Yet midwives are required to do so much that they are breaking, they cannot do much more. Calls for kindness, compassion, resilience and other virtues are addressed to midwives. Yet those midwives do not receive kindness and compassion and have scarcely time to smile and welcome each new client with whom they have fleeting, timed and closely programmed contact." (Kirkham 2019).

It is the economic and political structures which underpin the system that are the issue. I am not condoning poor practice or denying that it exists: the stories in this book illustrate that. But the problem is far deeper and, on the whole, blaming health care professionals and exhorting them to do things differently won't make a significant difference without wider cultural change.

But it's not appropriate to put the onus on woman and families themselves. As with some of the other issues of our time, such as climate change and what we eat, pressure is often put on individuals to make changes and take control of their destiny when the reality is that so much power lies in the hands of multinational companies and those who benefit from the capitalist, patriarchal ideas that have long permeated our culture. Can some women and families help themselves if they have better information? Yes, sometimes. That's why a lot of the work I do is about explaining evidence and putting information into readable formats so that people can better understand the issues and have that kind of information if they want to take it into account in making the decisions that are right for them. But the suggestion that we can and should all take control of our own destiny is itself part of the problem: many people do not have the privilege, the education, the resources or the support to be able to do this. Many women and families don't even know that there are other options, or that they have human rights when it comes to pregnancy and birth options and decisions.

Reframing normality, understanding risk

I do believe there is some hope, though. There are many examples, both in this book and elsewhere, of how women, midwives and others are reclaiming women's spaces, redefining normality and reframing conversations about risk (Murphy-Lawless 1998, Edwards & Murphy-Lawless 2006, Wickham 2008, 2011, Cheyne *et al* 2012, Reed 2019a, 2019b). Many people have come to realise that the current approach isn't logical, and are sharing their thoughts on this. These are important conversations, and we need to have more of them.

This reframing may be evidence of the fact that a revolution is underway, and by this I mean the kind of revolution that philosopher Thomas Kuhn (1962) discussed. Kuhn wrote about scientific revolutions, or changes in the ideas that a culture believes over time. He showed that the finding of anomalies – or things that don't fit the existing model – can lead to paradigm shifts. In fact, he coined the word paradigm. Some of the studies about induction and the challenges that I and others have raised could be said to be anomalies. That's because they clearly show that medical theories about birth in general and induction of labour in particular are wrong. It is in fact possible (and I acknowledge that this is an optimistic view, but I think optimism is vital in difficult times) that one reason that our culture feels so divided, polarised and tumultuous right now is because we are in the 'eye of the storm' in the middle of a paradigm shift.

One of the ideas that stems from my own work in this area (Wickham 2008) that I would urge everyone to think about is how western medicine often conflates pathology – by which we mean actual medical conditions, like pre-eclampsia, rhesus disease or a heart condition – with risk. But risk and pathology are two very different things. The vast majority of those who are deemed to be 'at risk' will never experience the problem that they or their health care providers are worried about. In this situation, the word 'risk' simply means 'chance.' It doesn't mean 'you have a medical condition.' Life itself is risky, and we all encounter risks every day. Getting out of bed is risky, but thankfully not very risky, so we generally all do this every morning. We need to put risks into context.

We also need to help people better understand risk. The concept of risk is used to scare people into compliance in many aspects of life. Yet, as I have shown in this book, there is little to no evidence to support routine induction of labour in the many groups of women who are being told they are 'at risk.' Even when there is some evidence showing that induction might be beneficial in certain situations if we look just at short-term outcomes, that evidence is often weak, and we would need to induce lots of women/babies (and thus expose them to the long-term risks of induction) in order to prevent one stillbirth. But remember that we don't know whether or how many other babies will pay a price for that in later life. We must also never forget that the downsides of induction may outweigh the possible benefits for the individual woman/family.

Living in our own time

As I've said throughout this book, there is no right or wrong answer when it comes to induction of labour. Medicine isn't a pure science, despite what some people claim. There are no absolutes or guarantees, whatever you do, and although it can seem hard to believe, our knowledge is actually very limited.

But my hope for you, now that you've reached the end of this book, is that you have a better understanding of why we have an induction epidemic. About how the idea of routine induction isn't really evidence-based and that the current, medicalised, technocratic approach to the end of pregnancy is only one approach, and not necessarily the right approach for everyone. If you're pregnant or thinking of becoming pregnant, I hope you'll feel more able to make the decisions that are right for you, and more able to help those around you to enjoy the end of their pregnancy more. I also hope you'll take some of the ideas in this book with you after you close it. There is value in reminding people that babies aren't like pumpkins and that due dates are better expressed as month-long windows.

It's also really important to remember that we are the descendants of thousands of generations of women who have successfully given birth. If you are pregnant, or planning a pregnancy, I want to also remind you that you are no less capable than your ancestors were. You may be living in a culture that wants you to think otherwise. The female body is really capable of growing, birthing and feeding a baby and, when we support ourselves and each other to do that, intervention isn't routinely needed. We need to do whatever we can to remind ourselves and others of that.

Let's continue to engage and work collectively to change the conversation and culture around pregnancy and birth, and also around other oppressive aspects of our lives and our world that are undermining community, sustainability and life itself.

It's vital that we recognise that many of the achievements of the past few hundred years have been beneficial, but that our current industrialised approach does harm as well as good. It's clear that we need to keep learning, questioning and talking; to unpack some of the ideas that we have become attached to, and come up with better ones. While not forgetting to look up at the moon now and again, just as our ancestors might have done, and wonder at the miracle that is birth and the fact that, in most cases, if we leave well alone, it happens at the right time.

If you have enjoyed this book and found it useful, please leave a review at your favourite book retailer – it really helps highlight it to others who might need it.

To see more of Sara's work:

Visit my website at www.sarawickham.com

Sign up for my free monthly newsletter and get information on new books, courses and projects at www.tinyurl.com/saranews

Other books by Sara which you might enjoy:

Anti-D Explained

Birthing Your Placenta: the third stage of labour

Inducing Labour: making informed decisions

Group B Strep Explained

Vitamin K and the Newborn

What's Right For Me? Making decisions in pregnancy and childbirth

101 tips for planning, writing and surviving your dissertation

References

ACOG (2021). Medically indicated late-preterm and early-term deliveries. O&G 138(1): 166-69.

Adler K, Rahkonen L, Kruit H (2020). Maternal childbirth experience in induced and spontaneous labour measured in a visual analog scale and the factors influencing it. BMC P&C 20(1):415.

Akuamoah-Boateng J & Spencer R (2018). Woman-centered care: Women's experiences and perceptions of induction of labor for uncomplicated post-term pregnancy: A systematic review of qualitative evidence. Midwifery 67: 46-56.

Alterman N, Johnson S, Carson C *et al* (2021). Gestational age at birth and child special educational needs: a UK representative birth cohort study. Arch Dis Childhood. doi: 10.1136/archdischild-2020-320213

Amis D (2014) Healthy Birth Practice #1: Let Labor Begin on Its Own. J Perinat Ed 23(4): 178–87.

Anderson T (2002). Out of the Laboratory: back to the darkened room. MIDIRS Midwifery Digest 12(1):65-69.

Anekwe L (2020). Ethnic disparities in maternal care BMJ 368:m442.

Ankarcrona V, Altman D, Wikström A-K *et al* (2019). Delivery outcome after trial of labor in nulliparous women 40 years or older - A nationwide population-based study. AOGS 98: 1195-1203.

Aune D, Saugstad OD, Henriksen T *et al* (2014). Maternal body mass index and the risk of fetal death, stillbirth, and infant death: a systematic review and meta-analysis. JAMA. 311(15):1536-46.

Ballantyne JW (1902). The problem of the postmature infant. JOG Brit Emp 2(36): 521-44.

Barrett A (2014). #Notallobstetricians https://dralisonbarrett.wordpress.com/2014/08/31/notallobstetricians/

Baskett TE & Allen AC (1995). Perinatal implications of shoulder dystocia. O&G 86: 14-17.

Baud D, Rouiller S, Hohlfeld P et al (2013). Adverse obstetrical and neonatal outcomes in elective and medically indicated inductions of labor at term. JM-FNM 26(16): 1595-1601.

Beech B (1987). Who's Having Your Baby? Surbiton: AIMS.

Bergholt T, Lim LK, Jorgensen JS et al (2007). Maternal body mass index in the first trimester and risk of cesarean delivery in nulliparous women in spontaneous labor. AJOG 196(2): e161-165.

Bergholt T, Skjeldestad FE, Pyykönen A et al (2020). Maternal age and risk of cesarean section in women with induced labor at term - A Nordic register-based study. AOGS 99: 283- 89.

Bergsjo P, Daniel W & Denman DW (1990). Duration of human singleton pregnancy; a population-based study. AOGS 69: 197-207.

Beta J, Khan N, Khalil A et al (2019). Maternal and neonatal complications of fetal macrosomia: a systematic review and meta-analysis. Ultrasound OG 54(3): 308-18.

Bhide A (2021). Induction of labor and caesarean section. AOGS 100(2): 187-88.

Birthplace in England Collaborative Group (2011). Perinatal and maternal outcomes by planned place of birth for healthy women with low risk pregnancies: the Birthplace in England national prospective cohort study. BMJ 343:d7400. doi.org/10.1136/bmj.d7400

Blackwell SC, Refuerzo J, Chadha R et al (2009). Overestimation of fetal weight by ultrasound: does it influence the likelihood of cesarean delivery for labor arrest? AJOG 200(3):340.e1-3.

Born C (2021). The Secret of Ishango – On the helix structure of prime numbers. AfricArXiv doi.org/10.31730/osf.io/yz6nq

Boulvain M, Irion O, Dowswell T *et al* (2016). Induction of labour at or near term for suspected fetal macrosomia. The Cochrane Database of Systematic Reviews. 10.1002/14651858.cd000938. pub2.

Boyle EM, Johnson S, Manktelow B *et al* (2015). Neonatal outcomes and delivery of care for infants born late preterm or moderately preterm. Arch Dis Child Fetal Neonatal Ed 100:F479–85.

Bricker L, Medley N, Pratt JJ *et al* (2015). Routine ultrasound in late pregnancy (after 24 weeks' gestation). Cochrane Database of Systematic Reviews 2015, Issue 6. Art. No.: CD001451.

Brigante L & Harlev-Lam B (2021). The RCM response to the NICE induction of labour draft guideline. www.rcm.org.uk/news-views/rcm-opinion/2021/the-rcm-response-to-the-nice-induction-of-labour-draft-guideline/

Brown SJ & Furber CM (2015). Women's experiences of cervical ripening as inpatients on an antenatal ward. Sex Rep Hlthc 6(4): 219-25.

Brown HK, Speechley KN, Macnab J *et al* (2014). Neonatal morbidity associated with late preterm and early term birth: the roles of gestational age and biological determinants of preterm birth. Int J Epid 43: 802–14.

Buckley SJ (2015). Hormonal Physiology of Childbearing: evidence and implications for women, babies, and maternity care. Washington DC: Childbirth Connection Programs, National Partnership for Women & Families.

Butler J, Abrams B & Parker J (1993). Supportive nurse-midwife care is associated with a reduced incidence of cesarean section. AJOG 168(5): 1407-13.

Çalik KY, Karabulutlu Ö & Yavuz C (2018). First do no harm - interventions during labor and maternal satisfaction: a descriptive cross-sectional study. BMC P&C 18(1): 1-10.

Cameron CM, Shibl R, McClure RJ *et al* (2014). Maternal pregravid BMI and child hospital admissions in the first 5 years of life: results from an Australian birth cohort. Int J Obesity 38(10): 1268-74.

Carlhäll S, Källén K & Blomberg M (2020). The effect of maternal body mass index on duration of induced labor. AOGS 99(5): 669-78.

Carlson NS, Corwin EJ & Lowe NK (2017). Labor intervention and outcomes in women who are nulliparous and obese: comparison of nurse-midwife to obstetrician intrapartum care. JMWH 62: 29-39.

Carolan M, Davey MA, Biro MA *et al* (2011). Older maternal age and intervention in labor: a population-based study comparing older and younger first-time mothers in Victoria, Australia. Birth, 38(1): 24–29.

Cartwright A (1979). The dignity of labour? A study of childbearing and induction. London: Tavistock.

Cerdeña JP, Plaisime MV & Tsai J (2020). From race-based to race-conscious medicine: how anti-racist uprisings call us to act. Lancet 396(10257): 1125-28.

Chan B & Lao T (2009). Maternal height and length of gestation: Does this impact on preterm labour in Asian women? ANZJOG 49: 388–92.

Chan E, Leong P, Malouf R *et al* (2016). Long-term cognitive and school outcomes of late-preterm and early-term births: a systematic review. Child Care Health Dev 42(3): 297-312.

Chauhan SP, Grobman WA, Gherman RA *et al* (2005). Suspicion and treatment of the macrosomic fetus. AJOG 193(2): 332-46.

Cheng ER, Declercq ER, Belanoff C *et al* (2015). Labor and delivery experiences of mothers with suspected large babies. MCHJ 19(12): 2578-86.

Cheyne H, Abhyankar P & Williams B (2012). Elective induction of labour: The problem of interpretation and communication of risks. Midwifery, 28(4): 412-415.

Clifford SH (1954). Postmaturity - with placenta dysfunction. J Ped 44:1.

Coates D, Donnollet N, Foureur M *et al* (2020a). Women's experiences of decision-making and attitudes in relation to induction of labour: A survey study. Women and Birth 34(2): e170-e177.

Coates D, Makris A, Catling C *et al* (2020b). A systematic scoping review of clinical indications for induction of labour. Plos One 15(1): e0228196.

Coates R, Cupples G, Scamell A *et al* (2018). Women's experiences of induction of labour: Qualitative systematic review and thematic synthesis. Midwifery. 69: 17-28.

Coates R, Cupples G, Scamell A *et al* (2021). Women's experiences of outpatient induction of labour with double balloon catheter or prostaglandin pessary: A qualitative study. Women & Birth 34(4) e406-15.

Coates R, McCourt C, Scamell M *et al* (2019). Induction of labour should be offered to all women at term. FOR: Induction of labour should be offered at term. BJOG doi.org/10.1111/1471-0528.16628.

Condon J, Jeyasuria P, Faust J *et al* (2004). Surfactant protein secreted by the maturing mouse fetal lung acts as a hormone that signals the initiation of parturition. Proceedings of the NAS USA. https://www.pnas.org/content/101/14/4978.full

Crequit S, Korb D, Morin C *et al* (2020). Use of the Robson classification to understand the increased risk of cesarean section in case of maternal obesity. BMC P&C 20(1): 738.

Dahlen H (2015). Being born is good for you. TPM. 18(4): 10-13.

Dahlen HG, Kennedy HP, Anderson CM *et al* (2013).The EPIIC hypothesis: Intrapartum effects on the neonatal epigenome and consequent health outcomes. Medical Hypotheses 80(5): 656-62.

Dahlen HG, Thornton C, Downe S *et al* (2021). Intrapartum interventions and outcomes for women and children following induction of labour at term in uncomplicated pregnancies: a 16-year population-based linked data study. BMJ Open 11:e047040.

Dalbye R, Gunnes N, Blix E *et al* (2021). Maternal body mass index and risk of obstetric, maternal and neonatal outcomes: A cohort study of nulliparous women with spontaneous onset of labor. AOGS 100: 521–30.

Davey M-A & King J (2016). Caesarean section following induction of labour in uncomplicated first births - a population-based cross-sectional analysis of 42,950 births. BMC P&C 16: 92.

Davies-Tuck M, Wallace EM & Homer CSE (2018). Why ARRIVE should not thrive in Australia. Women and Birth 31(5): 339-40.

Davis G, Waldman B, Phipps H *et al* (2021). A survey of obstetricians' attitudes to induction of labour at 39 weeks gestation with the intention of reducing caesarean section rates. ANZJOG 61: 94–99.

Davis-Floyd RE (1992). Birth as an American Rite of Passage. Berkeley: U. California Press.

Davis-Floyd RE (1993). The Technocratic Model of Birth. In: Hollis ST, Pershing L & Young MJ (1993). Feminist Theory in the Study of Folklore. Chicago: U. Illinois Press. 297-326.

Daviss BA and Johnson K (1998) Statistics and Research Committee [statistics on cervical ripening] MANA Newsletter, 16(2): 16-17.

Declercq ER, Sakala C, Corry MP *et al* (2007). Listening to mothers II: report of the second national US survey of women's childbearing experiences. J Perinat Ed 16(4): 9.

Declercq ER, Sakala C, Corry MP *et al* (2014). Major Survey Findings of Listening to Mothers(SM) III: Pregnancy and Birth: Report of the Third National U.S. Survey of Women's Childbearing Experiences. J Perinat Ed 23(1): 9-16.

Declercq ER, Belanoff C & Sakala C (2020). Intrapartum care and experiences of women with midwives versus obstetricians in the Listening to Mothers in California Survey. JMWH 65(1):45-55.

Denison FC, Aedla NR, Keag O *et al* (2018). Care of Women with Obesity in Pregnancy. Green-top Guideline No. 72. London: RCOG.

Denona B, Foley M, Mahony R *et al* (2020). Discrimination by parity is a prerequisite for assessing induction of labour outcome – cross-sectional study. *BMC Pregnancy Childbirth* 20: 709.

Derraik JG, Savage T, Hofman PL *et al* (2016). Shorter mothers have shorter pregnancies. JOG 36(1): 1-2.

de Vries BS, Barratt A, McGeechan K *et al* (2019). Outcomes of induction of labour in nulliparous women at 38 to 39 weeks pregnancy by clinical indication: An observational study. ANZJOG 59(4): 484-92.

Douglass C & Lokugamage A (2021). Racial profiling for induction of labour: improving safety or perpetuating racism? BMJ Blogs https://blogs.bmj.com/bmj/2021/10/15/racial-profiling-for-induction-of-labour-improving-safety-or-perpetuating-racism/

Downe S, Finlayson K, Oladapo OT et al (2018). What matters to women during childbirth: A systematic qualitative review. PLOS ONE 13(5): e0197791.

Drandić D & van Leeuwen F (2020). COVID-19: a watershed moment for women's rights in childbirth. Med Anth Quart 8(11).

D'Souza R, Horyn I, Jacob CE *et al* (2021). Birth outcomes in women with body mass index of 40 kg/m2 or greater stratified by planned and actual mode of birth. AOGS 100(2), 200-09.

Duan M, Wang Y, Zhang Q *et al* (2021) Characteristics of gut microbiota in people with obesity. PLoS ONE 16(8): e0255446.

Dupont C, Blanc-Petitjean P, Cortet M *et al* (2020). Dissatisfaction of women with induction of labour according to parity: results of a population-based cohort study. Midwifery 84: 102663.

Ebrahimoff M, Many A, Downe S *et al* (2020). Length of labour in mothers and their daughters: A matched cohort study. EJOGRB 245:77-83.

Edwards NP & Murphy-Lawless J (2006). The Instability of Risk: women's perspectives on risk and safety in birth. In: Symon, A(2006). Risk and choice in maternity care. Edinburgh: Churchill Livingstone.

Edwards N (2019). Birthing your baby: the second stage of labour. Edinburgh: BPPF.

El Marroun, Zou R, Leeuwenburg MF *et al* (2020). Association of gestational age at Birth With Brain Morphometry. JAMA Ped 174(12): 1149-58.

Elverdam B & Wielandt H (1994). The duration of a human pregnancy - medical fact or cultural tradition? Int J Prenat Perinat Psych & Med 6(2): 239-46.

Enkin M, Kierse MJNC, Neilson J *et al* (2000). A guide to effective care in pregnancy and childbirth. (Third edition). New York: OUP.

Espada-Trespalacios X, Ojeda F, Rodrigo NN *et al* (2021). Induction of labour as compared with spontaneous labour in low-risk women: A multicenter study in Catalonia. Sex Rep Health 29: 100648.

Everett, C (2017). Numbers and the Making of Us: Counting and the Course of Human Cultures. Boston: Harvard University Press.

Fang F, Zhang QY, Zhang J *et al* (2019). Risk factors for recurrent macrosomia and child outcomes. World J Pediatr 15(3): 289-96.

Figlio DN, Guryan J, Karbownik K *et al* (2016). Long-term cognitive and health outcomes of school-aged children who were born late-term vs full-term. JAMA Ped 170(8): 758-64.

Flenady V, Koopmans L, Middleton P *et al* (2011). Major risk factors for stillbirth in high-income countries: a systematic review and meta-analysis. Lancet 377(9774): 1331-40.

Flint SW & Reale S (2014). Obesity stigmatisation from obesity researchers. Lancet 384(9958): 1925-26.

Fuchs K & Wapner R (2006). Elective cesarean section and induction and their impact on late preterm births. Cl Perinat 33(4): 793-801.

Fyfe E, Anderson N, North R *et al* (2011). Risk of first-stage and second-stage cesarean delivery by maternal body mass index among nulliparous women in labor at term. O&G 117(6): 1315–22.

Gaskin IM (2004) Understanding birth and sphincter law. BJM 12(9): 540-42.

Gaudet L, Wen SW & Walker M (2014). The combined effect of maternal obesity and fetal macrosomia on pregnancy outcomes. JOGC 36(9): 776-84.

Gennser G, Ohrlander S & Eneroth P (1977). Fetal cortisol and the initiation of labour in the human. Ciba Found Symp. 47: 401-26.

Geronimus AT (1992). The weathering hypothesis and the health of African-American women and infants: evidence and speculations. Ethnicity & Disease. 2(3): 207-21.

Gibbons L, Belizán JM, Lauer JA *et al* (2010). The global numbers and costs of additionally needed and unnecessary caesarean sections performed per year: overuse as a barrier to universal coverage. World Health Rep Background Paper 30: 1-31.

Gill JV & Boyle EM (2017). Outcomes of infants born near term. Arch Dis Child 102(2): 194-98.

Giscombe CL & Lobel M (2005). Explaining disproportionately high rates of adverse birth outcomes among African Americans: the impact of stress, racism, and related factors in pregnancy. Psychol Bull 131(5): 662-83.

Glantz JC (2019). Elective Induction at 39 Weeks of Gestation and the Implications of a Large, Multicenter, Randomized Controlled Trial. O&G 134(1): 178-79.

Glazer KB, Danilack VA, Field AE *et al* (2020). Term labor induction and cesarean delivery risk among obese women with and without comorbidities. A J Perinat doi: 10.1055/s-0040-1714422.

Goer H (2018). Preventive Induction of Labor: Does Mother Nature Know Best? https://www.lamaze.org/Connecting-the-Dots/Post/preventive-induction-of-labor-does-mother-nature-know-best-henci-goer-examines-the-arrive-study

Goyal NK, Attanasio LB & Kozhimannil KB (2014). Hospital care and early breastfeeding outcomes among late preterm, early-term, and term infants. Birth 41: 330–38.

Grobman WA, Rice MM, Reddy UM *et al* (2018). Labor induction versus expectant management in low-risk nulliparous women. NEJM 379: 513-23.

Gross TL, Sokol RJ, Williams T *et al* (1987). Shoulder dystocia: a fetal-physician risk. AJOG 156: 1408–18.

Gunnarsdóttir J, Swift EM, Jakobsdóttir J *et al* (2021). Cesarean birth, obstetric emergencies, and adverse neonatal outcomes in Iceland during a period of increasing labor induction. Birth 10.1111/birt.12564

Haavisto H, Polo-Kantola P, Anttila E *et al* (2021). Experiences of induction of labor with a catheter. A prospective randomized controlled trial comparing the outpatient and inpatient setting. AOGS 100(3): 410-17.

Hall ET (1984). The dance of life: the other dimension of time. New York: Anchor Press.

Hamm RF, Teefey CP, Dolin CD *et al* (2021). Risk of cesarean delivery for women with obesity using a standardized labor induction protocol. A J Perinat DOI: 10.1055/s-0041-1732459

Harkness M, Yuill C, Cheyne H *et al* (2021). Induction of labour during the COVID-19 pandemic: a national survey of impact on practice in the UK. BMC P&C 21: 310.

Hasseljo R & Auberg AC (1962). Prolonged pregnancy. AOGS 61: S23-S29.

Helman Cl (1987). Heart disease and the cultural construction of time. Social Science & Medicine 25(9): 969-79.

Henderson J & Redshaw M (2013). Women's experience of induction of labor: a mixed methods study. AOGS 92(10): 1159-67.

Heys S, Downe S & Thomson G (2021). 'I know my place'; a meta-ethnographic synthesis of disadvantaged and vulnerable women's negative experiences of maternity care in high-income countries. Midwifery 103, in press. doi.org/10.1016/j.midw.2021.103123.

Hildingsson I, Karlström A & Nystedt A (2011). Women's experiences of induction of labour - findings from a Swedish regional study ANZJOG 51(2): 151-57.

Homer CSE, Leap N, Edwards N *et al* (2017). Midwifery continuity of carer in an area of high socio-economic disadvantage in London: A retrospective analysis of Albany Midwifery Practice outcomes using routine data (1997–2009). Midwifery 48: 1-10.

HSIB (2020). Severe brain injury, early neonatal death and intrapartum stillbirth associated with larger babies and shoulder dystocia. London: HSIB.

Huang L, Sauve R, Birkett D *et al* (2008). Maternal age and risk of stillbirth: a systematic review. CMAJ 178(2): 165-72.

Iacobucci G (2020). Obesity: medical leaders call for end to "stigmatising" language. BMJ 368 :m858.

Inch S (1982). Birthrights: A parents' guide to modern childbirth. London: Hutchinson.

Jevitt CM, Stapleton S, Deng Y *et al* (2021). Birth outcomes of women with obesity enrolled for care at freestanding birth centers in the United States. JMWH 66: 14-23.

Johantgen M, Fountain L, Zangaro G *et al* (2012). Comparison of labor and delivery care provided by certified nurse-midwives and physicians: a systematic review, 1990 to 2008. WHI 22(1): e73-e81.

Jones C & Jomeen J (2017). Women with a BMI ≥ 30kg/m² and their experience of maternity care: A meta ethnographic synthesis. Midwifery 53: 87-95.

Jukic AM, Baird DD, Weinberg CR *et al* (2013). Length of human pregnancy and contributors to its natural variation. Hum Reprod 28(10): 2848-55.

Källén B, Finnström O, Nygren K-G *et al* (2013). Maternal and fetal factors which affect fetometry: use of in vitro fertilization and birth register data. EJOGRB 170: 372–76.

Katz Rothman B (1982). In Labour. Women and Power in the Birthplace. London: Junction Books.

Katz Rothman B (1984). Giving Birth: Alternatives in Childbirth. New York, Penguin.

Kawakita T, Iqbal SN, Huang C-C *et al* (2017). Nonmedically indicated induction in morbidly obese women is not associated with an increased risk of cesarean delivery. AJOG 217(4):451.e1–.e8.

Kenyon S, Skrybant M, Johnston T *et al* (2019). Optimising the management of late term pregnancies. BMJ 364:l681.

Kerrigan A, Kingdon C & Cheyne H (2015). Obesity and normal birth: a qualitative study of clinician's management of obese pregnant women during labour. BMC P&C 15(256).

Keulen JKJ, Bruinsma A, Kortekaas JC *et al* (2018). Timing induction of labour at 41 or 42 weeks? A closer look at time frames of comparison: A review. Midwifery 66: 111-18.

Keulen JKJ, Nieuwkerk PT, Kortekaas JC *et al* (2020). What women want and why. Women's preferences for induction of labour or expectant management in late-term pregnancy. Women and Birth 34(3): 250-56.

Khambalia AZ, Roberts CL, Nguyen M *et al* (2013). Predicting date of birth and examining the best time to date a pregnancy. IJGO 123(2): 105-09.

King BC, Hagan J, Suresh G *et al* (2019). The effects of labor induction at 39 weeks in low-risk nulliparous women. Acta Paediatrica 108(5): 974.

Kirkham M (2017). A Fundamental Contradiction: the business model does not fit midwifery values. Midwifery Matters 152: 13-15.

Kirkham M (2019). Midwives should… https://www.birthpractice andpolitics.org/post/2019/10/02/midwives-should

Kitzinger S (2006). Birth Crisis. London: Routledge.

Kitzinger S (1987). Freedom and Choice in Childbirth. Penguin.

Kjerulff KH, Attanasio LB, Edmonds JK *et al* (2017). Labor induction and cesarean delivery: A prospective cohort study of first births in Pennsylvania, USA. Birth 44: 252-61.

Knight HE, Cromwell DA, Gurol-Urganci I *et al* (2017). Perinatal mortality associated with induction of labour versus expectant management in nulliparous women aged 35 years or over: An English national cohort study. PLOS Medicine 14(11): e1002425.

Knight M, Bunch K, Tuffnell D *et al* on behalf of MBRRACE-UK (2018). Saving Lives, Improving Mothers' Care - Lessons learned to inform maternity care from the UK and Ireland Confidential Enquiries into Maternal Deaths and Morbidity 2014-16. Oxford: NPEU.

Knight M, Bunch K, Tuffnell D *et al* on behalf of MBRRACE-UK (2020). Saving Lives, Improving Mothers' Care - Lessons learned to inform maternity care from the UK and Ireland Confidential Enquiries into Maternal Deaths and Morbidity 2016-18. Oxford: NPEU.

Knight-Agarwal CR, Williams LT, Davis D (2016). The perspectives of obese women receiving antenatal care: A qualitative study of women's experiences. Women and Birth 29(2): 189-95.

Kominiarek MA, Vanveldhuisen P, Hibbard J *et al* (2010). Consortium on Safe Labor. The maternal body mass index: a strong association with delivery route. AJOG 203(03): 264.e1–264.e7.

Kortekaas JC, Kazemier BM, Keulen JKJ *et al* (2020). Risk of adverse pregnancy outcomes of late- and postterm pregnancies in advanced maternal age: A national cohort study. AOGS 99: 1022–30.

Kuhn TS (1962). The Structure of Scientific Revolutions. U Chicago Press.

Kullinger M, Haglund B, Kieler H *et al* (2016). Effects of ultrasound pregnancy dating on neonatal morbidity in late preterm and early term male infants. BMC P&C 16(1): 1-8.

Lanman JT (1968). Delays during reproduction and their effects on the embryo and fetus. NEJM 278: 1092-99.

Lavecchia M, Sabbah M & Abenhaim HA (2018). Effect of planned mode of delivery in women with advanced maternal age. MCHJ 20(11): 2318-27.

Lawson GW (2021). Naegele's rule and the length of pregnancy – A review. ANZJOG 61(2): 177-82.

Lee V, Darney B, Snowden J *et al* (2016). Term elective induction of labour and perinatal outcomes in obese women: retrospective cohort study. BJOG 123(2): 271–78.

Lee I-M, Shiroma EJ, Kamada M *et al* (2019). Association of step volume and intensity with all-cause mortality in older women. JAMA Intern Med 179(8): 1105-12.

Leung T, Stuart O, Suen S *et al* (2011). Comparison of perinatal outcomes of shoulder dystocia alleviated by different type and sequence of manoeuvres: a retrospective review. BJOG 118: 985-90.

Levine EM, Delfinado LN, Locher S *et al* (2021). Reducing the Cesarean Delivery Rate. EJOGRB 262: 155-59.

Li Y, Townend J, Rowe R *et al* (2014). The effect of maternal age and planned place of birth on intrapartum outcomes in healthy women with straightforward pregnancies: secondary analysis of the Birthplace national prospective cohort study. BMJ Open 4(1): e004026.

Lie RT, Wilcox A, Skjaerven R (2006). Maternal and paternal influences on length of pregnancy. O&G 107(4): 880-85.

Lightly K & Weeks A (2020). Authors' reply re: Induction of labour should be offered to all women at term. BJOG 128: 935-36.

Little J, Nugent R & Vangaveti V (2019). Influence of maternal obesity on Bishop Score and failed induction of labour: A retrospective cohort study in a regional tertiary centre. ANZJOG 59: 243-50.

Loftin RW, Habli M, Snyder CC *et al* (2010). Late preterm birth. Rev O&G 39(1), 10–19.

Lokugamage AU, Rix E, Fleming T *et al* (2021). Translating Cultural Safety to the UK. J Med Ethics doi: 10.1136/medethics-2020-107017.

Lothian JA (2006). Saying "No" to Induction. J Perin Ed. 15(2): 42-45.

Lou S, Hvidman L, Uldbjerg N *et al* (2019). Women's experiences of postterm induction of labor: A systematic review of qualitative studies. Birth 46(3): 400-10.

Lutsiv O, Giglia L, Pullenayegum E *et al* (2013). A population-based cohort study of breastfeeding according to gestational age at term delivery. J Pediatr 163: 1283–88.

Machin D & Scamell M (1997). The experience of labour using ethnography to explore the irresistible nature of the bio-medical metaphor during labour. Midwifery 13(2): 78-84.

Main EK, Chang S-C, Cheng Y *et al* (2020). Hospital-level variation in the frequency of cesarean delivery among nulliparous women who undergo labor induction. O&G 136(6): 1179-89.

Mander R (2013). Induction of labour for advancing maternal age. EM 4(8): 46-49.

Marmot M, Allen J & Boyce T (2020). Health equity in England: the Marmot review 10 years on. BMJ 2020;368: m693.

Marrs C, La Rosa M, Caughey A *et al* (2019). In Reply. Obstet Gynecol 134(1): 179. doi: 10.1097/AOG.0000000000003343.

Mathews TJ & MacDorman MF (2013). Infant mortality statistics from the 2010 period linked birth/infant death data set. NCHS. www.cdc.gov/ nchs/data/nvsr/nvsr62/nvsr62_08.pdf

McAlpine JM, Scott R, Scuffham PA *et al* (2016). The association between third trimester multivitamin/mineral supplements and gestational length in uncomplicated pregnancies. Women and Birth 29(1): 41-46.

Middleton P, Shepherd E, Morris J *et al* (2020). Induction of labour at or beyond 37 weeks' gestation. Cochrane Database of Systematic Reviews 2020, Issue 7. Art. No.: CD004945. DOI: 10.1002/14651858.CD004945.pub5.

Miller S, Abalos E, Chamillard M *et al* (2016). Beyond too little, too late and too much, too soon: a pathway towards evidence-based, respectful maternity care worldwide. Lancet 388(10056): 2176-92.

Milner J & Arezina J (2018). The accuracy of ultrasound estimation of fetal weight in comparison to birth weight: A systematic review. Ultrasound. 26(1): 32-41.

Ministry of Health (1970). Domiciliary Midwifery and Maternity Bed Needs: the Report of the Standing Maternity and Midwifery Advisory Committee (Sub-committee Chairman J. Peel). HMSO, London.

Mittendorf R, Williams MA & Berkey, CS (1990). The length of uncomplicated human gestation. O&G 75: 929-32.

Mittendorf R, Williams MA & Berkey CS (1993). Predictors of human gestational length. AJOG 168: 480-84.

Mogren I, Stenlund H, Högberg U (1999). Recurrence of prolonged pregnancy. Int J Epid 28(2): 253-57.

Moraitis AA, Shreeve N, Sovio U *et al* (2020). Universal third-trimester ultrasonic screening using fetal macrosomia in the prediction of adverse perinatal outcome: A systematic review and meta-analysis of diagnostic test accuracy. PLOS Med 17(10): e1003190.

Morken N-H, Melve K, Skjaerven R (2011). Recurrence of prolonged and post-term gestational age across generations: maternal and paternal contribution. BJOG 118: 1630–35.

Muglu J, Rather H, Arroyo-Manzano D *et al* (2019). Risks of stillbirth and neonatal death with advancing gestation at term: A systematic review and meta-analysis of cohort studies of 15 million pregnancies. PLoS Med 16(7): e1002838.

Murphy-Lawless J (1998). Reading Birth and Death: A history of obstetric thinking. Cork University Press.

Murphy-Lawless J (2018). Responding to the tragedy of maternal health: A collective challenges the state. In: Edwards N, Mander R & Murphy-Lawless J (2018). Untangling the Maternity Crisis. Routledge.

Naegele K (1830). Lehrbuch der Geburtshilfe für Hebammen. Heidelberg.

Nagahawatte NT & Goldenberg RL (2008). Poverty, maternal health, and adverse pregnancy outcomes. Annals NY Acad Sci 1136: 80-85.

Nath RK, Avila MB, Melcher SE *et al* (2015). Birth weight and incidence of surgical obstetric brachial plexus injury. Eplasty 15:e14.

Neel A, Cunningham CE & Teele GR (2021). A routine third trimester growth ultrasound in the obese pregnant woman does not reliably identify fetal growth abnormalities: A retrospective cohort study. ANZJOG 61: 116-22.

Nelson KB, Sartwelle TP & Rouse DJ (2016). Electronic fetal monitoring, cerebral palsy, and caesarean section: assumptions versus evidence. BMJ 2016; 355: i6405.

Ng KYB & Steer PJ (2016). Prediction of an estimated delivery date should take into account both the length of a previous pregnancy and the interpregnancy interval. EJOGRB 201: 101-07.

NICE (2008a). Induction of Labour. London, RCOG.

NICE (2008b). Antenatal care for uncomplicated pregnancies. London: NICE.

NICE (2021a). National Institute for Health and Care Excellence Guideline: Inducing Labour. Draft for consultation. May 2021. London: NICE.

NICE (2021b). National Institute for Health and Care Excellence Guideline: Inducing Labour. November 2021. London: NICE.

Noble KG, Fifer WP, Rauh VA *et al* (2012). Academic achievement varies with gestational age among children born at term. Pediatrics 130(2): e257–e264.

Oakley A (1980). Women Confined, Towards a Sociology of Childbirth. Oxford: Martin Robertson.

Oakley A (1984). The Captured Womb. Oxford: Blackwell.

Oakley A (1993). Essays on Women, Medicine and Health. Edinburgh University Press.

Oberg AS, Frisell T, Svensson AT *et al* (2013). Maternal and fetal genetic contributions to postterm birth: familial clustering in a population-based sample of 475,429 Swedish births. AJ Epid 177(6): 531-37.

Olsen O (2019). Statistical analysis in SWEPIS trial is flawed. https://www.bmj.com/content/367/bmj.l6131/rapid-responses

Omigbodun A & Adewuyi A (1997). Duration of human singleton pregnancies in Ibadan, Nigeria. J Nat Med Assoc 89: 617–621.

Padmanabhan T & Padmanabhan V (2019). The Dawn of Science. Glimpses from History for the Curious Mind. Springer Nature.

Paluch AE, Gabriel KP, Fulton JE *et al* (2021). Steps per day and all-cause mortality in middle-aged adults in the coronary artery risk development in young adults study. JAMA Net Open 4(9): e2124516.

Papiernik E, Alexander G & Paneth N (1990). Racial differences in pregnancy duration and its implications for perinatal care. Med Hypotheses 33: 181– 86.

Pasupathy D, Wood AM, Pell JP *et al* (2011). Advanced maternal age and the risk of perinatal death due to intrapartum anoxia at term. J Epidemiol Community Health 65: 241–45.

Patel R, Steer P, Doyle P *et al* (2003). Does gestation vary by ethnic group? A London-based study of over 122,000 pregnancies with spontaneous onset of labour. Int J Epidem 33: 107–13.

Peleg D, Warsof S, Wolf MF *et al* (2015). Counseling for fetal macrosomia: an estimated fetal weight of 4,000 g is excessively low. Am J Perinatol. 32(1): 71-4.

Pickens C, Gibbs M, Kramer MR *et al* (2018). Term elective induction of labor and pregnancy outcomes among obese women and their offspring. O&G 131(1): 12–22.

Porter M & Macintyre S (1984). What is, must be best: a research note on conservative or deferential responses to antenatal care provision. Soc Sci Med 19(11): 1197-200.

Razai MS, Kankam HKN, Majeed A *et al* (2021). Mitigating ethnic disparities in covid-19 and beyond. BMJ 2021;372: m4921.

RCOG (2012a). Green top Guideline 42: Shoulder Dystocia. London: RCOG.

RCOG (2012b). In Vitro Fertilisation: Perinatal Risks and Early Childhood Outcomes. Scientific Impact Paper 8. London: RCOG.

RCOG (2013). Induction of labour at term in older mothers. London: RCOG.

Reed R (2018). Why induction matters. London: Pinter and Martin.

Reed R (2019a). Post-Dates Induction of Labour: balancing risks https://midwifethinking.com/2016/07/13/induction-of-labour-balancing-risks/

Reed R (2019b) Big Babies: the risk of care provider fear. https://midwifethinking.com/2019/09/02/big-babies-the-risk-of-care-provider-fear/

Relph S, Ong M, Vieira MC *et al* (2020). Perceptions of risk and influences of choice in pregnant women with obesity. An evidence synthesis of qualitative research. PLoS ONE 15(1): e0227325.

Relph S, Guo Y, Harvey ALJ *et al* (2021). Characteristics associated with uncomplicated pregnancies in women with obesity: a population-based cohort study. *BMC Pregnancy Childbirth* 21(182).

Roberts J, Evans K, Spiby H *et al* (2020). Women's information needs, decision-making and experiences of membrane sweeping to promote spontaneous labour. Midwifery 83: 102626.

Rosser J (2000). Calculating the EDD; which is more accurate, scan or LMP? TPM 3(3): 28-29.

Rossi AC, Mullin P & Prefumo F (2013). Prevention, management, and outcomes of macrosomia: a systematic review of literature and meta-analysis. Obstet Gynecol Surv. 68(10): 702-09.

Rouse DJ, Owen J, Goldenberg RL *et al* (1996). The effectiveness and costs of elective cesarean delivery for fetal macrosomia diagnosed by ultrasound. JAMA. 276(18): 1480-86.

Rowe R, Knight M, Kurinczuk JJ on behalf of the U.K. Midwifery Study System (UKMidSS) (2018). Outcomes for women with BMI> $35kg/m^2$ admitted for labour care to alongside midwifery units in the UK: A national prospective cohort study using the UK Midwifery Study System (UKMidSS). PLoS One. 13(12): e0208041.

Ruhstaller K (2015). Induction of labor in the obese patient. Semin Perinatol 39(6): 437-40.

Rui-Xue D, Xiu-Jie H & Chuan-Lai H (2019). The Association between Advanced Maternal Age and Macrosomia: A Meta-Analysis. Childhood Obesity 15:3.

Rydahl E, Declerq E, Juhl M *et al* (2019). Routine induction in late-term pregnancies: follow-up of a Danish induction of labour paradigm. BMJ Open 9:12.

Rydahl E, Eriksen L & Mette J (2019) Effects of induction of labour prior to post-term in low-risk pregnancies: a systematic review JBI Database System Rev Implement Rep 17(2): 170-208.

Saccone G, Della Corte L, Maruotti GM *et al* (2019). Induction of labor at full-term in pregnant women with uncomplicated singleton pregnancy: A systematic review and meta-analysis of randomized trials. AOGS 98: 958–66.

Sadeh-Mestechkin D, Walfisch A, Shachar R *et al* (2008). Suspected macrosomia? Better not tell. Arch GO 278(3): 225-30.

Sakala C, Declercq ER, Corry MP (2002). Listening to Mothers: the first national U.S. survey of women's childbearing experiences. JOGNN 31(6): 633-34.

Sandall J, Soltani H, Gates S *et al* (2016). Midwife-led continuity models versus other models of care for childbearing women. Cochrane Database Syst Rev. 2016;(4):CD004667.

Sandall J, Tribe R, Avery L *et al* (2018). Short-term and long-term effects of caesarean section on the health of women and children. Lancet 392(10155): 1349-57.

Saunders N & Paterson C (1991). Can we abandon Naegele's rule? Lancet 337: 600-01.

Scialli A (2019a). Induction of labor at term. AJOG 221(1): 79.

Scialli AR (2019b). Elective Induction at 39 Weeks of Gestation and the Implications of a Large, Multicenter, Randomized Controlled Trial O&G 134(1):177-78.

Schwarz C, Gross MM, Heusser P *et al* (2016). Women's perceptions of induction of labour outcomes: results of an online-survey in Germany. Midwifery, 35: 3-10.

Seife C (2000). Zero: The biography of a dangerous idea. London: Souvenir Press.

Seijmonsbergen-Schermers AE, Scherjon S & De Jonge A (2019). Induction of labour should be offered to all women at term: AGAINST: Induction of labour should not be offered to all women at term: first, do no harm. BJOG 126 (2019): 1599.

Seijmonsbergen-Schermers AE, Peters LL, Goodarzi B *et al* (2020). Which level of risk justifies routine induction of labor for healthy women? Sexual and Reproductive Healthcare 23: 100479.

Shallow H (2019). Is induction of labour morally justifiable? https://www.birthpracticeandpolitics.org/post/2019/03/25/is-induction-of-labour-morally-justifiable

Simons RL, Lei MK, Beach SRH *et al* (2016). Economic hardship and biological weathering: the epigenetics of aging in a U.S. sample of black women. Soc Sci Med 150:192–200.

Sjöö M & Mor B (1991). The Great Cosmic Mother: Rediscovering the Religion of the Earth. San Fransisco: HarperCollins.

Small K (2020). Are doctors still improving childbirth? www.birthsmalltalk.com/2020/11/05/are-doctors-still-improving-childbirth/

Smith GC (2001). Use of time to event analysis to estimate the normal duration of human pregnancy. Hum Reprod 16(7): 1497-1500.

Souter V, Painter I, Sitcov K et al (2019a). Maternal and newborn outcomes with elective induction of labor at term. AJOG 220(3): 273.e1-11.

Souter V, Nethery E & Kopas ML (2019b). Comparison of midwifery and obstetric care in low-risk hospital births. O&G 134(5): 1056-65.

Speert H (1958). Essays in eponymy. New York, Macmillan.

Stene-Larsen K, Lang AM, Landolt MA *et al* (2016). Emotional and behavioral problems in late preterm and early term births: outcomes at child age 36 months. BMC Pediatr 16(1): 196.

Stickler GB (1994). Expected date of confinement (correspondence). J Family Practice 39(4): 325.

Studelska J (2012). The last days of pregnancy: A place of in-between. Mothering. April 9, 2012.

Tew M (1985). Place of birth and perinatal mortality. JRCGP 35 (277): 390-94.

Tew M (1986). Do obstetric intranatal interventions make birth safer? BJOG 93(6): 659-74.

Tew M (1998). Safer childbirth: a critical history of maternity care. Third edition. London: Free Association Books.

Timpka S & Larsson J (2019). On the early termination of the SWEPIS trial. https://www.bmj.com/content/367/bmj.l6131/rr

Todd AL, Zhang LY, Khambalia AZ *et al* (2017). Women's views about the timing of birth. Women and Birth 30(2): e78-e82.

Treasure J & Ambwani S (2021). Addressing weight stigma and anti-obesity rhetoric in policy changes to prevent eating disorders. Lancet 398(10294): 7-8.

Treloar A, Behn B & Cowan D (1967a). Analysis of gestational interval. AJOG 99: 34–45.

Treloar A, Boynton R, Behn B *et al* (1967b). Variation of the human menstrual cycle through reproductive life. Int J Fertil 12: 77–126.

Unicef (2021). Research on skin-to-skin contact. www.unicef.org.uk/babyfriendly/newsandresearch/babyfriendlyresearch/research-supporting-breastfeeding/skin-to-skin-contact/

van der Kooy B (1994). Calculating expected date of delivery - its accuracy and relevance. Midwifery Matters 60: 4-7, 24.

van Teijlingen E (2005) A critical analysis of the medical model as used in the study of pregnancy and childbirth. Sociological Research Online 10(2).

van Teijlingen ER, Hundley V, Rennie A-M *et al* (2003). Maternity satisfaction studies and their limitations: "What is, must still be best". Birth 30(2): 75-82.

Wagner M (2006). Born in the USA. How a broken maternity system must be fixed to put women and children first. Berkeley: U Cal Press.

Walker KF, Bugg GJ, Macpherson M *et al* (2016a). Randomized trial of labor induction in women 35 years of age or older. NEJM 374(9): 813-22.

Walker KF, Bradshaw L, Bugg GJ *et al* (2016b). Causes of antepartum stillbirth in women of advanced maternal age. EJOGRB 197: 86-90.

Wang Y, Tanbo T, Abyholm T *et al* (2011). The impact of advanced maternal age and parity on obstetric and perinatal outcomes in singleton gestations. AGO 284(1): 31–37.

Warland J & Mitchell EA (2014). A triple risk model for unexplained late stillbirth. BMC P&C 14: 142.

Warwick Clinical Trials Unit (2021). Induction of labour for predicted macrosomia - The 'Big Baby Trial. www.warwick.ac.uk/fac/sci/ med/research/ctu/trials/bigbaby

Wastlund D, Moraitis AA, Thornton JG *et al* (2019). The cost-effectiveness of universal late-pregnancy screening for macrosomia in nulliparous women: a decision analysis. BJOG 126(10): 1243-50.

Weiss E, Krombholz K & Eichner M (2014). Fetal mortality at and beyond term in singleton pregnancies in Baden-Wuerttemberg/Germany 2004–2009. Arch Gyn Obstetrics 289(1): 79-84.

Wennerholm UB, Hagberg H, Brorsson B *et al* (2009). Induction of labor versus expectant management for post-date pregnancy: is there sufficient evidence for a change in clinical practice? AOGS 88: 6-17.

Wennerholm U, Saltvedt S, Wessberg A *et al* (2019). Induction of labour at 41 weeks versus expectant management and induction of labour at 42 weeks (SWEdish Post-term Induction Study, SWEPIS): multicentre, open label, randomised superiority trial. BMJ 367 :l6131.

Whitworth M, Bricker L, Mullan C (2015). Ultrasound for fetal assessment in early pregnancy. Cochrane Database Syst Rev (7): CD007058.

Wickham S (2008). An exploration of holistic midwives' knowledge in relation to "post-term" pregnancy. Unpublished PhD thesis.

Wickham S (2009a). Stepping stones and cervical wisdom. Birthspirit Midwifery Journal 3: 39-42. Available on www.sarawickham.com

Wickham S (2009b). Post-term pregnancy: the problem of the boundaries. MIDIRS Midwifery Digest 19 (4): 463-9.

Wickham S (2011). Stretching the fabric: from technocratic normal limits to holistic midwives' negotiations of normalcy. EM 2(11): 17-23. Available on www.sarawickham.com

Wickham S (2014). Does induction really reduce the likelihood of caesarean section? TPM 17(8): 39-40.

Wickham S (2016). Questioning induction of labour in older women. TPM 19(7): 36-37. Available on www.sarawickham.com

Wickham S (2018a). Inducing labour: making informed decisions. Avebury: Birthmoon Creations.

Wickham S (2018b). What's right for me? Making decisions in pregnancy and childbirth. Avebury: Birthmoon Creations.

Wickham S (2019). Group B Strep Explained. Avebury: Birthmoon Creations.

Wickham S (2020). Membrane sweeping for induction of labour https://www.sarawickham.com/research-updates/membrane-sweeping-for-induction-of-labour/

Wickham S (2021). How to cancel an induction https://www.sarawickham.com/riffing-ranting-and-raving/how-to-cancel-a-labour-induction/

Wickham S & Robinson D (2010). Nil nocere: doing no harm as an important guiding principle within maternity care. MIDIRS Midwifery Digest 20(4): 415-20. Available on www.sarawickham.com

Wolfe H, Timofeev J, Tefera E *et al* (2014). Risk of cesarean in obese nulliparous women with unfavorable cervix: elective induction vs expectant management at term. AJOG 211(1):53.e1–5.

Wolrich J (2021). Food isn't medicine. London: Vermilion.

Woolner AMF & Bhattacharya S (2015). Obesity and stillbirth. Best Pract Res Clin Obstet Gynaecol 29(3): 415-26.

Zaslavsky C (1979). Africa Counts: Number and Pattern in African Culture. Chicago: L Hill.

Zaslavsky C (1991). Women as the first mathematicians. WME Newsletter 14(1): 4.

Zenzmaier C, Pfeifer B, Leitner H *et al* (2021). Cesarean delivery after non-medically indicated induction of labor: A population-based study using different definitions of expectant management. AOGS 100(2): 220-28.

Zhang J, Bricker L, Wray S *et al* (2007). Poor uterine contractility in obese women. BJOG 114(3): 343-48.

Zhao Y, Flatley C & Kumar S (2017). Intrapartum intervention rates and perinatal outcomes following induction of labour compared to expectant management at term from an Australian perinatal centre. ANZJOG 57(1): 40-48.

Also by Sara Wickham

Anti-D Explained

Anti-D is a medicine made from blood that is offered to rhesus negative women who may have been exposed to rhesus positive blood, for example as their baby is being born. Anti-D Explained helps parents and professionals to understand the science, the issues and the evidence relating to Anti-D.

Inducing Labour: making informed decisions

Sara's bestselling book explains the process of induction of labour and shares information from research studies, debates and women's, midwives' and doctors' experiences to help women and families get informed and decide what is right for them.

Group B Strep Explained

A popular book which helps parents, professionals and others to understand the issues and the evidence relating to the screening and prophylactic measures offered in the hope of preventing early-onset group B strep (EOGBS) disease.

Vitamin K and the Newborn

Find out everything you need to know about vitamin K; why it's offered to newborn babies, why are there different viewpoints on it and what do parents need to know in order to make the decision that is right for them and their baby?

What's Right For Me? Making decisions in pregnancy and childbirth

The decisions that we make about our childbirth journeys can shape our experiences, health and lives, and those of our families. A guide to the different approaches that exist; offering information, tips and tools to help you make the decisions that are right for you.

Also by Sara Wickham

Birthing Your Placenta (with Nadine Edwards)

A popular book which helps parents, professionals and others to understand the process and the evidence relating to the birth of the placenta. No matter what kind of birth you are hoping for, this book will help you understand the issues and options.

101 tips for planning, writing and surviving your dissertation

These 101 tips are useful for students at any stage of their academic career. Written in an accessible, friendly style and seasoned with first-hand advice, this book combines sound, practical tips from an experienced academic with reminders of the value of creativity, chocolate and naps in your work.

Printed in Great Britain
by Amazon